GUIDE TO THE RECOGNITION OF PIG DISORDERS

Copyright © 2019 Grupo Asís Biomedia, SL
Plaza Antonio Beltrán Martínez nº 1, planta 8 - letra I
(Centro empresarial El Trovador)
50002 Zaragoza - Spain

First printing: December 2019

Illustrator:
Jacob Gragera Artal

ISBN: 978-84-17640-34-7
DL: Z 2090-2019

Design, layout and printing:
Servet editorial - Grupo Asís Biomedia, SL
www.grupoasis.com
info@grupoasis.com

Servet is the publishing house of Grupo Asís

Warning:
Veterinary science is constantly evolving, as are pharmacology and the other sciences. Inevitably, it is therefore the responsibility of the veterinary surgeon to determine and verify the dosage, the method of administration, the duration of treatment and any possible contraindications to the treatments given to each individual patient, based on his or her professional experience. Neither the publisher nor the author can be held liable for any damage or harm caused to people, animals or properties resulting from the correct or incorrect application of the information contained in this book.

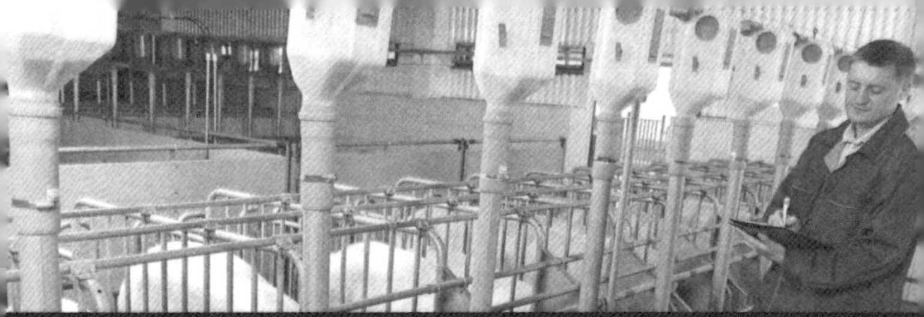

GUIDE TO THE RECOGNITION OF PIG DISORDERS

John Carr

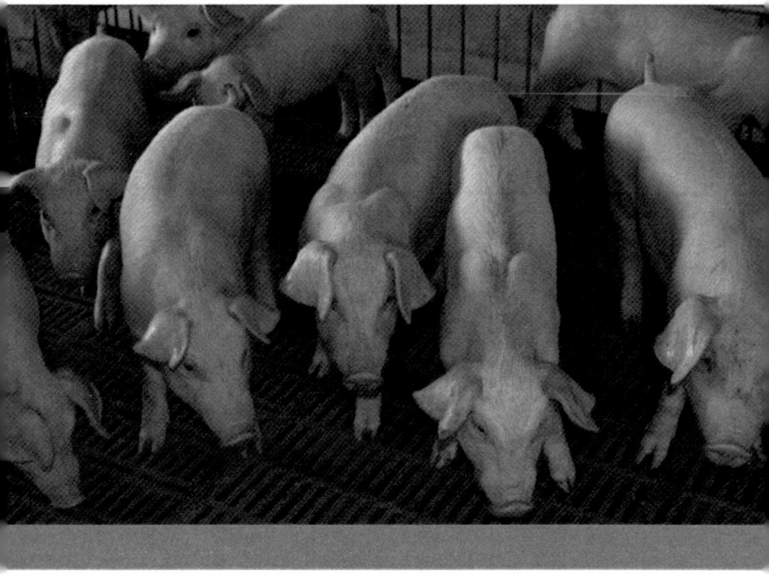

SERVET

THE AUTHOR

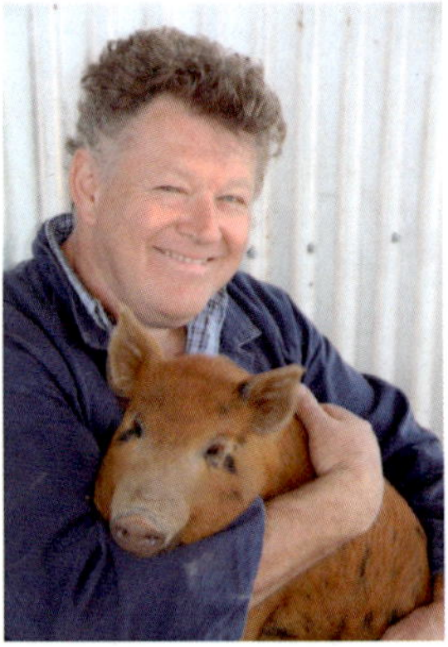

Dr. John Carr

Dr. Carr started learning the ropes about pigs at the age of 11. He qualified as a veterinarian in 1982 by the University of Liverpool. After 5 years in general practice he returned to university to complete a Leverhulme residency in pigs and a PhD in urinary tract problems of pigs at Liverpool, where he specialised in microbiology and pathology.

He has taught production medicine to veterinarians and farmers throughout the world through positions at several universities in the UK -Liverpool and Royal Veterinary College, London, and in the US -North Carolina and Iowa State- and in Western Australia at Murdoch and at James Cook University in Queensland.

Dr. Carr runs a consultancy practice with clients in North America, Europe, Asia, Australia and Africa. John specialises in maintaining the health of pigs through promoting excellence in stockmanship and production practices while controlling the cost of production. He has published several books and more than 200 refereed and non refereed articles.

PREFACE

The creatures outside looked from pig to man, and from man to pig, and from pig to man again; but already it was impossible to say which was which (George Orwell, Animal Farm, Ch. 10).

Welcome to *Guide to the Recognition of Pig Disorders.*

I hope you will find this guide useful and that it will enhance the health, welfare and wellbeing of your pigs.

The guide is written as an easy resource for veterinary practitioners, farmers and students of veterinary and animal science. For practicing advisors, it is a quick guide and a potential source of practical advice sheets for use on and around the farm.

The guide is aimed to provide information for the health of all pigs, from the single pet pig to large farms where pigs provide a vital protein source for humans.

The guide aims to provide information for the entire farm health team.

It aims to bring a more holistic approach to pig health management. The farm team should realise that the pig has changed little since its domestication and we need to farm according to the needs of the pig and not only to the needs of the stockperson.

The guide offers an introduction to the major disorders of the pig and provides a guide recognising these important diseases of pigs.

John Carr

TABLE OF CONTENTS

1

CLINICAL EXAMINATION SKILLS AND RECOGNITION OF PIG DISORDERS

INTRODUCTION

MAKING A DIAGNOSIS

A successful veterinarian is the one whose clients have no sick or compromised animals – an extremely difficult achievement. The clinician has to remember that final clinical signs are only the terminal cause of death. It is imperative that the veterinarian concentrates on maintaining the animal's health rather than treating its diseases.

MAKING AN ACCURATE DIAGNOSIS IS THE KEY TO SUCCESSFUL VETERINARY PRACTICE

A diagnosis is to identify:

- If there is a problem.
- The cause of the problem.
- Practical solutions to the problem.
- Means of preventing the problem occurring again.

IS THERE A PROBLEM?

In population medicine there are 6 essential key areas in assisting the clinician to make a diagnosis:

1. Taking a history of the problem.
2. The examination of the individual pig.
3. Postmortem examination of the individual pig.
4. Examination of the group of pigs.
5. Examination of the environment of the pig.
6. Examination of the farm performance.

Once the diagnosis has been made, this allows the vet to suggest practical solutions to the identified problem.

Taking a history of the problem

Clinicians have two ears and one mouth and should therefore listen twice as much as they talk.

Listening to the client and asking the correct questions is an essential component of making a diagnosis.

Consider the following line of enquiry:

What has the client seen? →	Is the pig eating, defecating, urinating, coughing, sneezing, lame or dying?
Severity of the problem? →	How many are sick or dead?
Location of the problem? →	Which pens or age groups are affected?
When did the problem start? →	Time, date, place?
How is the problem progressing? →	Are more pigs getting sick within the group?
More than one problem? →	How many different problems are there in the same group?
Epidemiological consideration? →	Has the problem spread to other groups?
Are there any other factors? →	Which factors does the client thinks are relevant to the situation?
What has the client done? →	Action to alleviate the problem? What was the result of the action?

The examination of the individual pig

In general practice a detailed individual examination of a pig is rarely performed, but it is essential to know the basics.

- Basic pig breeds.
- Basic pig terms.
- Handling and movement of pigs.
- Orientation around a pig.
- Surface anatomy of a pig.
- Weight and age of the pig, expected growth curve.
- Taking a blood sample from a pig (weaner and adult).
- Clinical examination of a cooperative and an uncooperative pig.
- Recognition and description of visible lesions.
- Auditing the welfare of the pig.

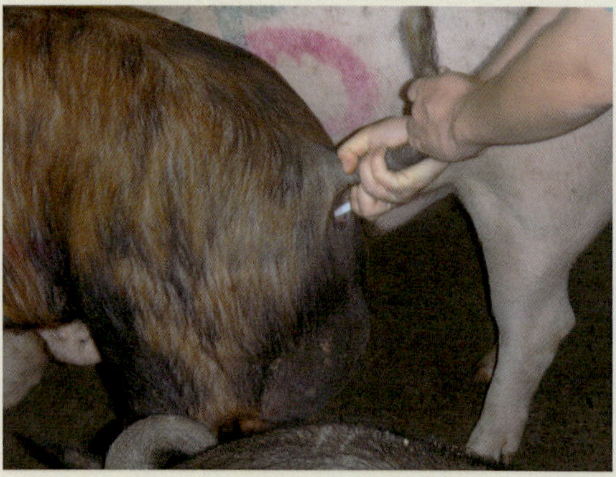

Figure 1. Taking the rectal temperature of a pig.

Postmortem technique

In population medicine the postmortem examination is a cornerstone to health maintenance. The postmortem routine needs to be methodical, to determine the likely cause of death of the individual. The veterinarian is also interested in the clinically relevant presence or absence of other specific pathogens.

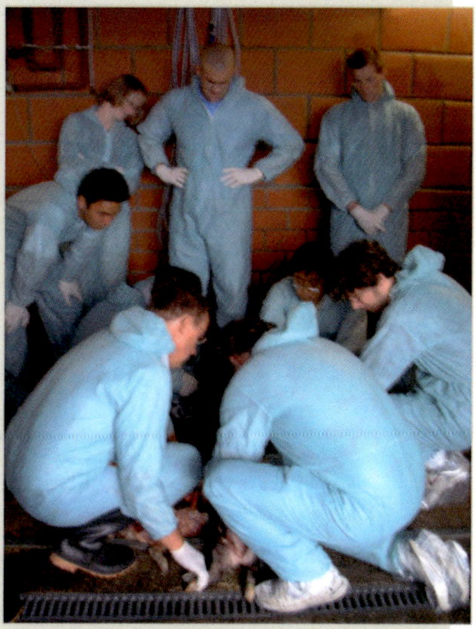

Figure 2. A farm team carrying out a postmortem examination.

Examination of the group of pigs

- Examination of the undisturbed group.
- Examination of the disturbed group.
- Examination of the farm.

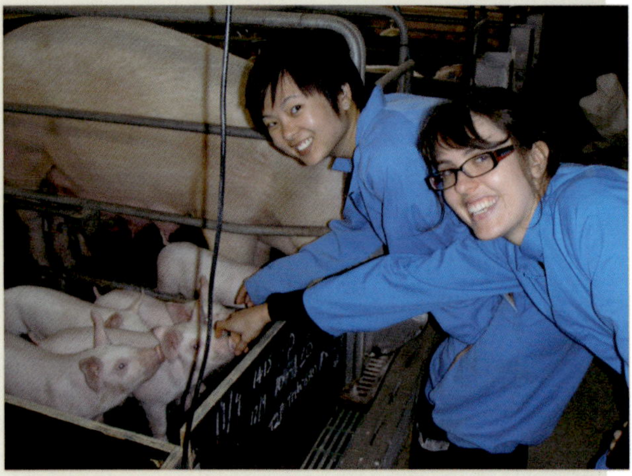

Figure 3. Examination of a group of pigs.

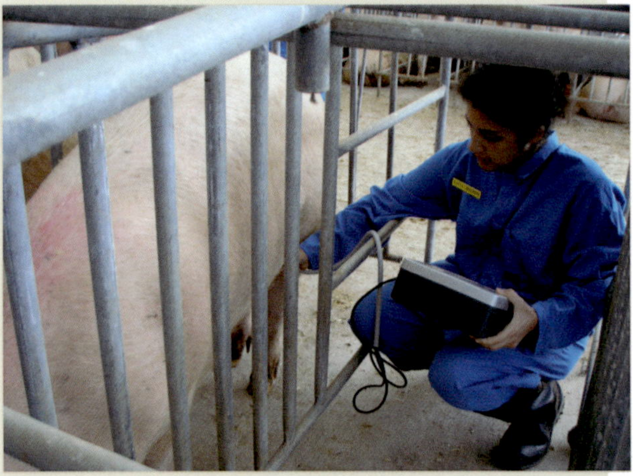

Figure 4. Carrying out an ultrasound pregnancy diagnosis.

Examination of the environment of the pig

You will be expected to know how to measure and record:

WATER	Type of drinker; height; flow and associated animal expectations
FOOD	Feeder space; feeder type; quantity of feed and basic make up of the feed
FLOOR	Space and stocking density, impact of worn equipment
AIR	Ventilation patterns, temperature, humidity and gas concentration expectations

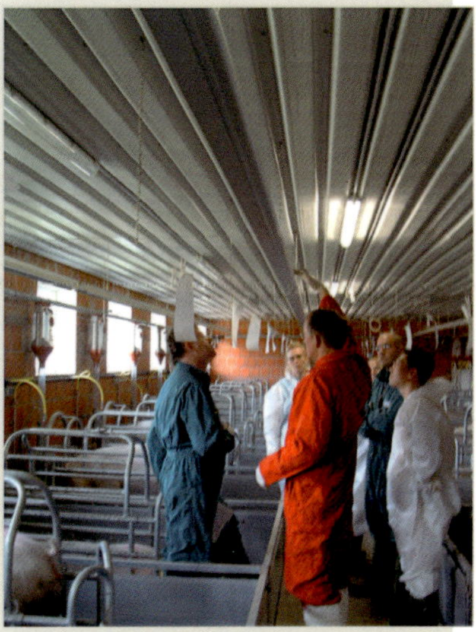

Figure 5. Examination of the ventilation system.

Examination of the farm performance

In any production system, a systematic approach is required to analyse any farm records.

CLINICAL EXAMINATION SKILLS

RECOGNITION OF CLINICAL SIGNS

Know what is normal about pigs – if you don't know what is normal, how can you recognise abnormal?

BEFORE ENTERING THE PEN

Look

Pig not eating

Pigs generally love food and a change in their eating patterns should always be a cause of further investigation.

Change in behaviour

- Depending on the group size, individual behaviours or the group's behaviour patterns may be known.
- Ideally, the stockperson will know all the pigs personally, even in a large group; however, individual pigs tend to stand out, whereas the mass, are sadly unknown. The animals that do stand out are the extremes – the top social order pigs, the lower social pigs and perhaps a few others who have unusual body markings – wolf pig, leopard spotted, etc.

Group behaviours

- Lying patterns
  Try to observe the known pigs and note their lying patterns and position within the group. A sow standing at 2.00 in the afternoon while all her companions are asleep is exhibiting an unusual behaviour and may be in heat (oestrus).
- Individual pig behaving differently
  - Look for pigs who are separated from the group.
  - See how groups of pigs behave when gathered around a drinker or a feeder.

▶

Listen

Note noises such as coughing or sneezing

- On entry to the room, observe the greeting sounds pigs make. Pigs with swine influenza are often very quiet and reluctant to stand up as you enter. Well-managed pigs should be pleased to see you.
- As pigs move around, note any coughing or sneezing.

Smell

Become familiar with the normal body odour of pigs. Swine dysentery and swine fever may cause malodorous smells.

ENTER AND MOVE AROUND THE PEN

Look

Look for the individuals, give them memorable names.

Movement

- Ensure all pigs stand up.
- Pigs can be stiff when rising, but within 5 to 10 strides, the stiffness should wear off.
- Walk over to any pigs who fail to rise up or walk off any stiffness.

Urination

When pigs rise up, particularly in the morning, they will urinate within 5 minutes. Note the colour of the urine and the posture of the pig urinating.

Blood

Look for any blood on the floor or walls.

Floor

Look at the floor for the consistency of stools (faeces).

Listen

As pigs move around, check for any coughing or sneezing.

Smell

Smell the air – if a pig has died the first indication may be a smell.

INDIVIDUAL PIG BEHAVIOR

- This includes any pig placed in a hospital pen.
- Pigs housed in small numbers should all be given names. This should include artificial insemination centres and adults on farms of less than 50 sows.

Know

Behaviour

Note any sudden or progressive change in pig's normal behaviour.

Feed

Know what food the pig likes and dislikes.

Reproduction

- Know what stage of reproduction the pig is at and note if the expected oestrus behaviour patterns fail to materialise.
- Changes in males (even when castrated) can occur in the presence of receptive females.

Look

- Loss of appetite – pigs should beg for food.
- Changes in behaviour – aggressive/less aggressive.
- Changes in head/ear posture.
- Changes in eye brightness.
- Change in skin colour or hair position.
- Locomotor changes – reluctance to stand up, do normal tricks.
- Dirty anal/tail area – diarrhoea. Changes in stools (faeces).
- Signs of vomiting.

Listen

Coughing, sneezing, wheezing and depth of breathing.

Feel

Presence of lumps – may be felt rather than seen

Once you have identified that there may be a problem, examine the pig in more detail.

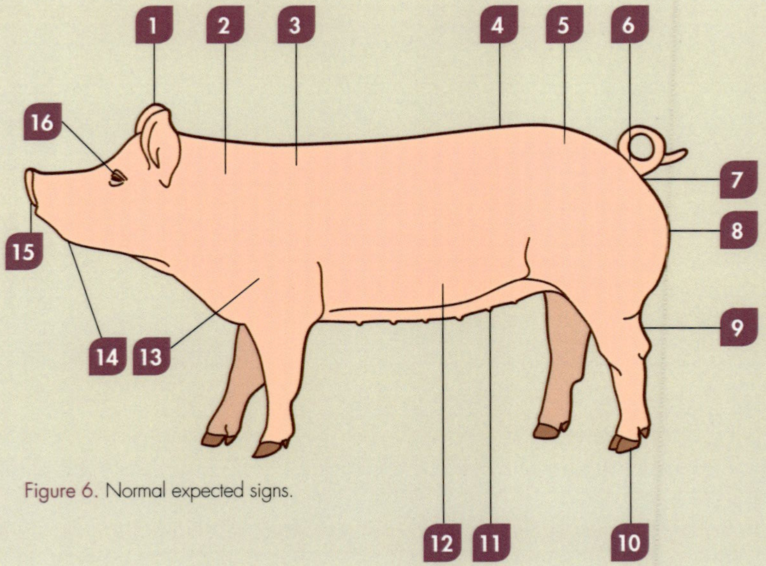

Figure 6. Normal expected signs.

1. Ears: raised, pointed at you.
2. Neck: no marks.
3. Hair: smooth, flat
4. Back: straight, meaty.
5. Hindquarters: meaty, smooth.
6. Tail "mood": alert, dip.
7. Anus: no faeces.
8. Vulva/testes: no discharge, small size.
9. Joints: no swelling easy movement.
10. Feet: even on ground, no swelling, marks or ulcers.
11. Mammary gland: no swelling, cold, even, full.
12. Belly: full, pregnant no swellings.
13. Chest: shallow, regular breathing.
14. Mouth: no discharge, no dropping of food.
15. Nose: raised sniffing.
16. Eyes: alert, bright.

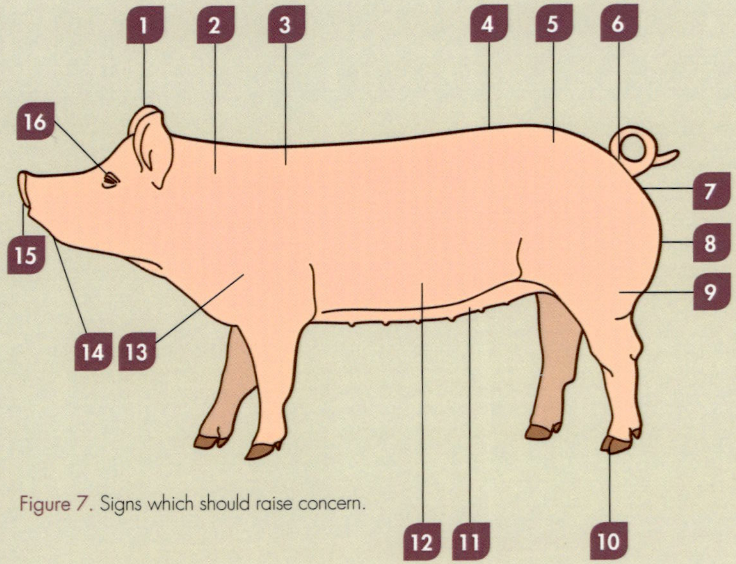

Figure 7. Signs which should raise concern.

1. Ears: droppy, discharge, lesions, necrosis, bite marks.
2. Neck: fighting, greasy pig.
3. Hair: raised, rough, irregular.
4. Back thin, wasting.
5. Hindquarters: uneven, lame, swelling, bite marks.
6. Tail: bitten, twitching, agitated.
7. Anus: diarrhoea, constipation.
8. Vulva/testes: discharge, swelling, coloured, deformed.
9. Joints: swelling, ulcer, lame, hot, pressure sores, trauma.
10. Feet: lame, ulcers, wounds, swelling, uneven cracks.
11. Mammary gland: swelling, heat, no milk, teat injuries.
12. Belly: empty, gaunt, swellings, kicking at it.
13. Chest: heave line, coughing, breathing rate, wheezing.
14. Mouth: discharge, food at mouth, deviation, salivation, tongue.
15. Nose: ulcer, discharge, running, sneezing, deviation.
16. Eyes: discharge, dehydration, conjunctivitis.

CLINICAL EXAMINATION OF THE INDIVIDUAL PIG – COOPERATIVE AND UNCOOPERATIVE

FOLLOW A SET PROCEDURE WHEN EXAMINING THE ANIMAL

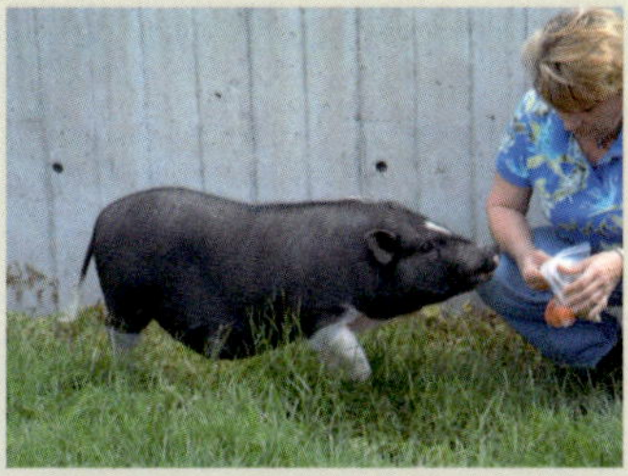

Figure 8. Assess the pig's normal behaviour, its locomotion and its response to its owners. Enquire about eating, urinating and defecating patterns.

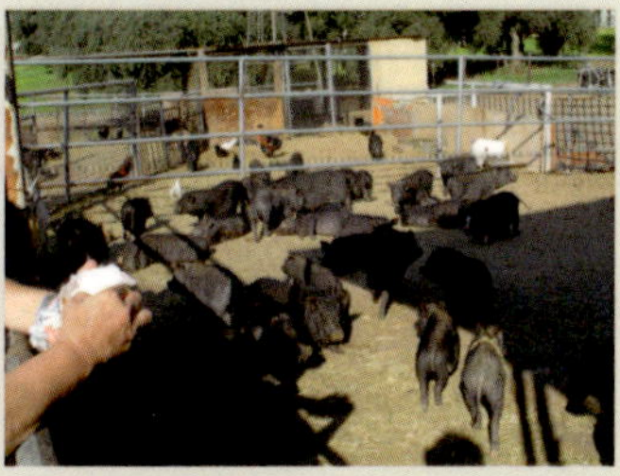

Figure 9. Remember the pig may live in a group and other pigs may be presenting with the same clinical signs.

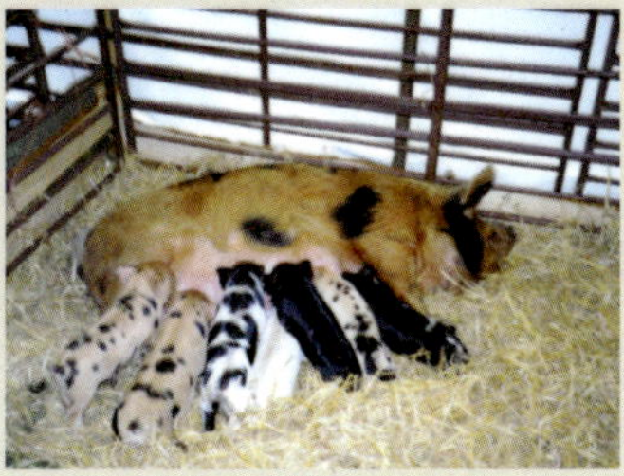

Figure 10. Enquire about the recent history of the pig.

EXAMINATION OF A COOPERATIVE PIG

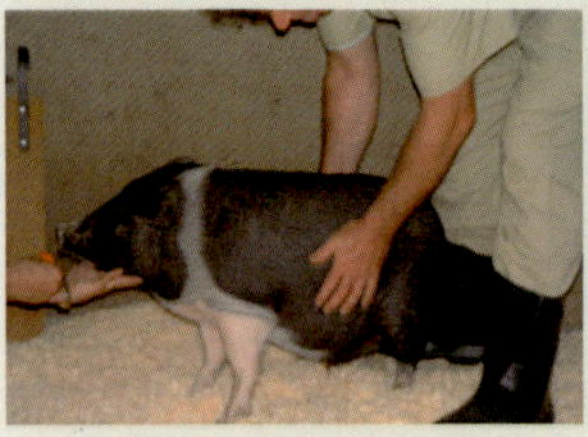

Figure 11. Make contact both vocally and physically. Assess body condition. Check breathing rate.

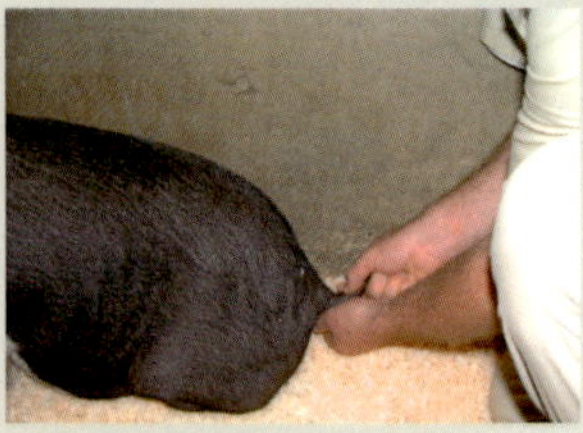

Figure 12. Take rectal temperature. Normal 39 °C. Examine the external genitalia.

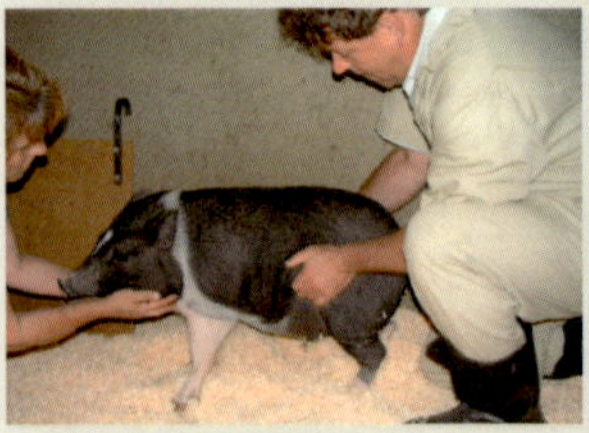

Figure 13. Palpate lumbar muscles, hind legs, abdomen and mammary area.

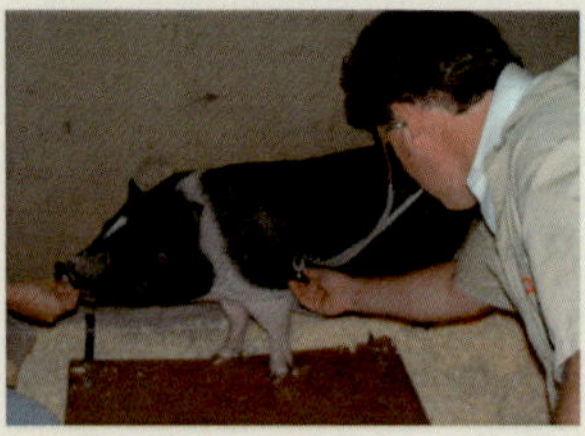

Figure 14. Some pigs may allow auscultation – but this is generally unrewarding.

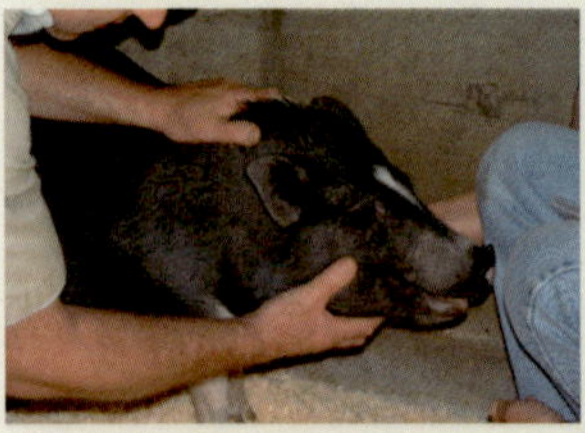

Figure 15. Pigs like being scratched particularly behind the ear and along the back. Check the head of the pig for any discharges from the nose, ears, eyes and mouth.

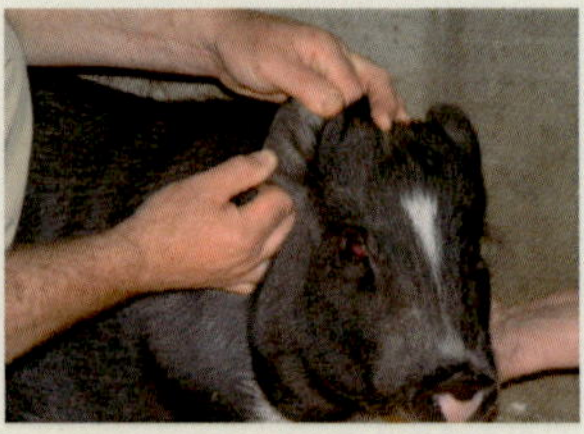

Figure 16. When handling the head, beware of the pig trying to bite.

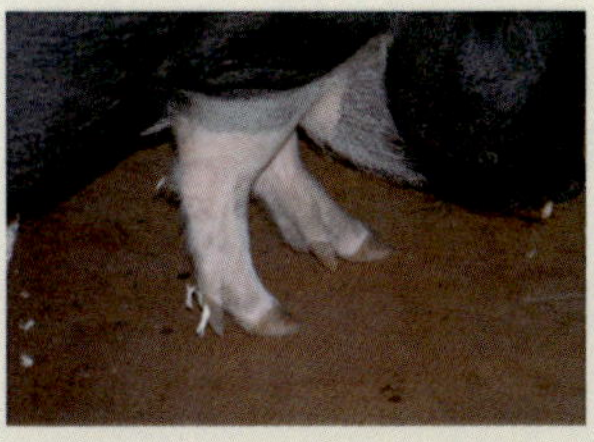

Figure 17. Examine the feet while standing.

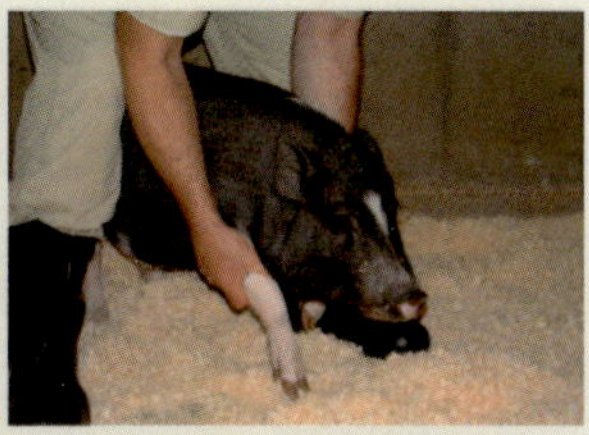

Figure 18. Grasp the pig's front legs firmly. The pig is likely to vocally object.

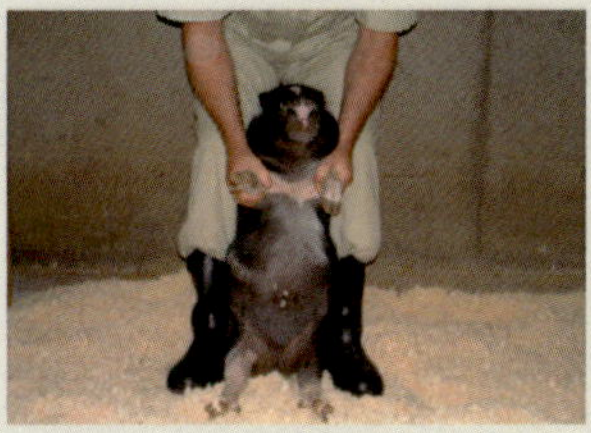

Figure 19. Place the pig on its rear, holding its back with your knees.

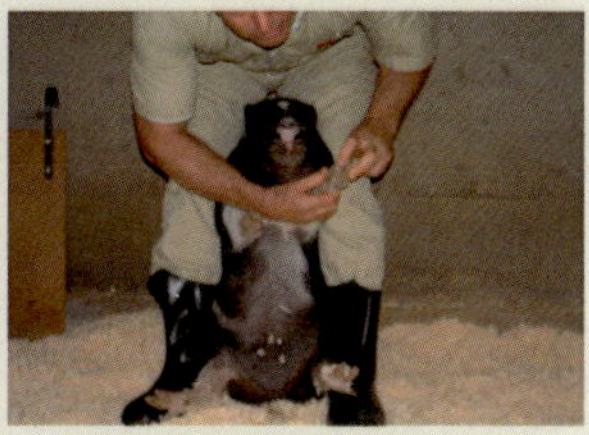

Figure 20. Palpation of the limbs should start at the top and work down the limb to the feet.

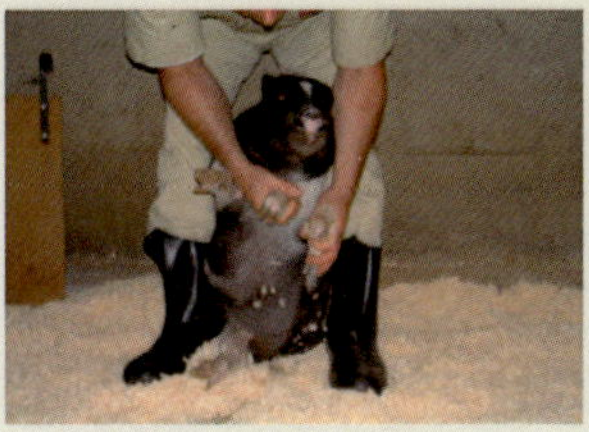

Figure 21. Palpation of the limbs should start at the top and work down the limb to the feet.

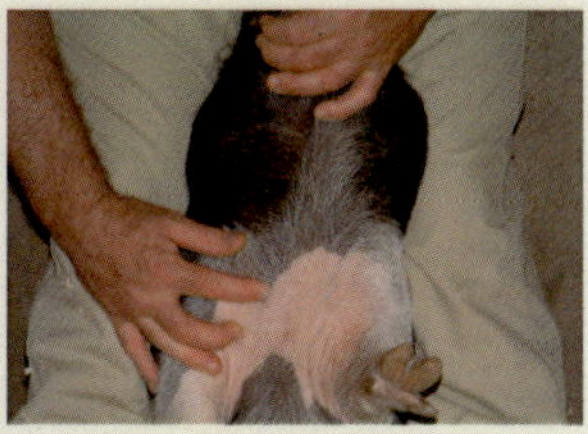

Figure 22. Collect any samples that are required. A blood sample can be obtained from the jugular vein in this sitting position.

EXAMINATION OF A UNCOOPERATIVE PIG

In an uncooperative pig, restrain the pig on its back from the sitting position where it will generally stop struggling.

A full clinical examination can now be completed starting from the rear to the front of the pig.

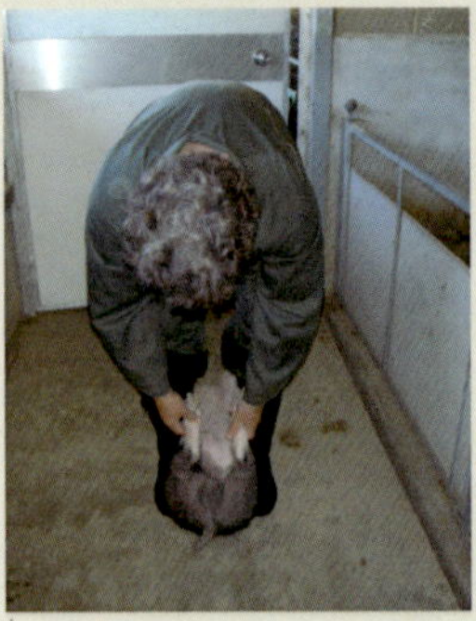

Figure 23. Walk backwards and lower the pig between your legs. Support its back with your feet and lower leg.

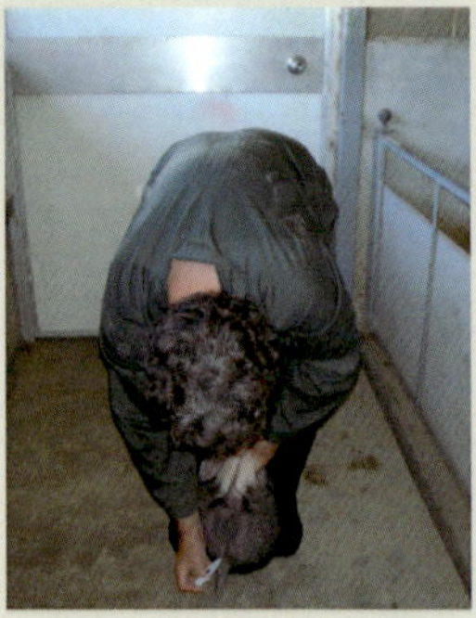

Figure 24. Keep a hold on the back legs and take the pig's rectal temperature.

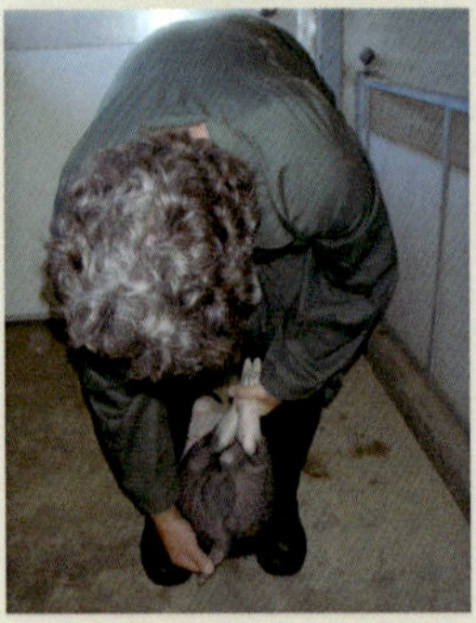

Figure 25. Examine the anus for any discharge. Take samples if necessary.

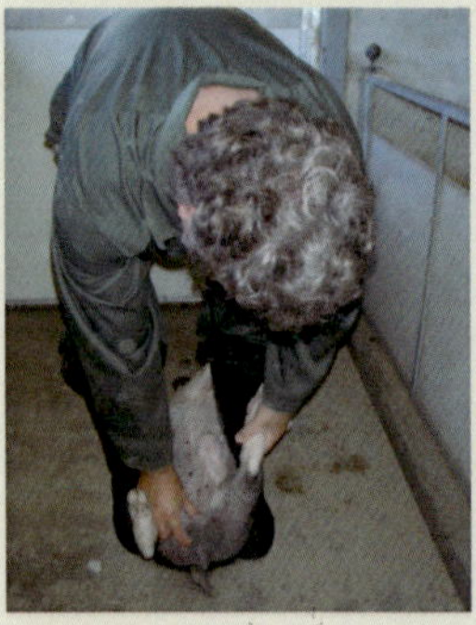

Figure 26. Examine the external genitalia.

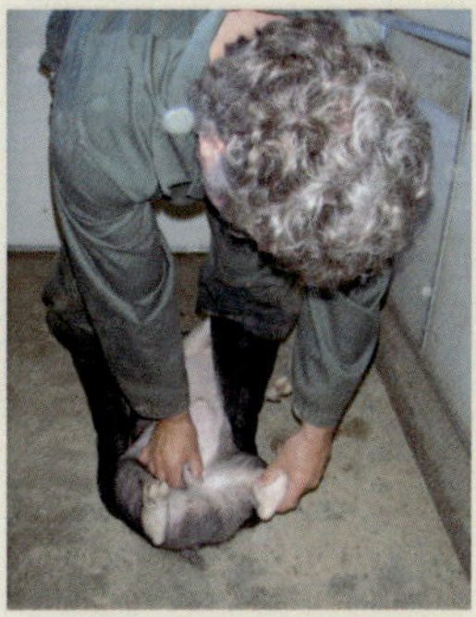

Figure 27. Examine the superficial lymph nodes.

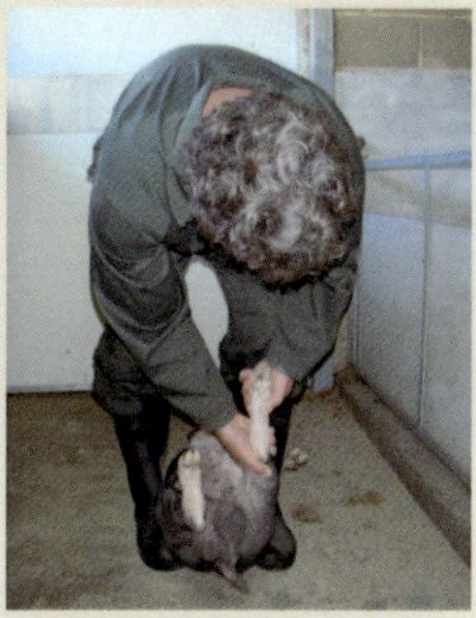

Figure 28. Examine the left hind leg from toe to hip.

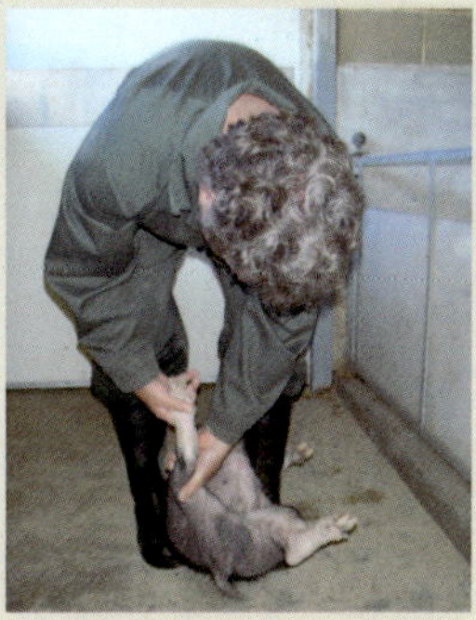

Figure 29. Examine the right hind leg from toe to hip.

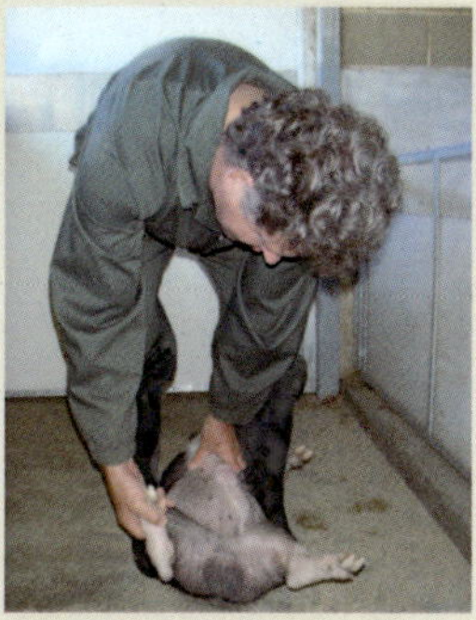

Figure 30. Examine the caudal ventral body wall and mammary glands.

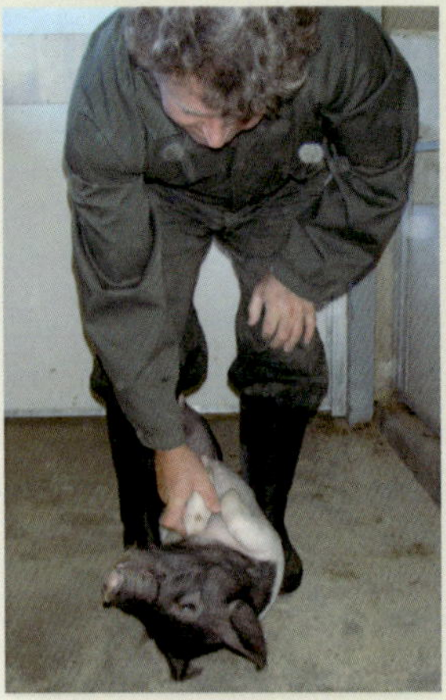

Figure 31. Carefully move or rotate your body to face the pig's head.

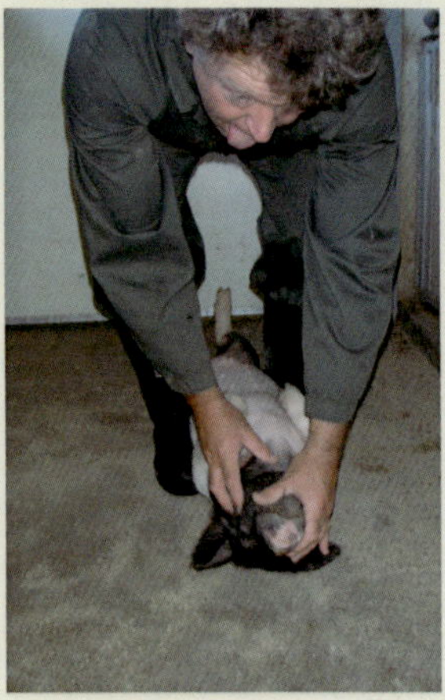

Figure 32. Support the pig with your feet under the shoulder blades.

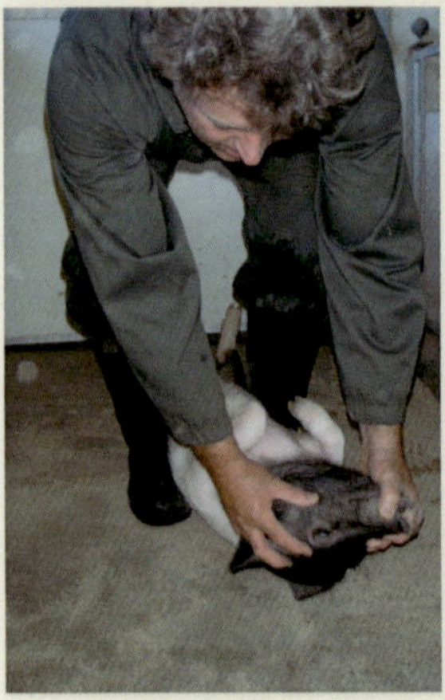

Figure 33. Examine the pig's eyes and jaw.

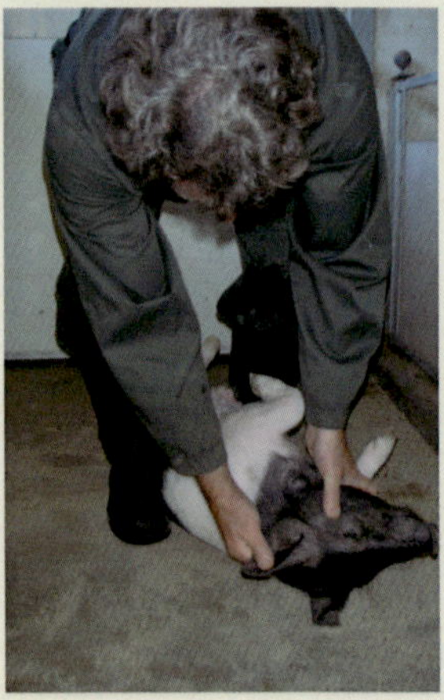

Figure 34. Examine the pig's ears.

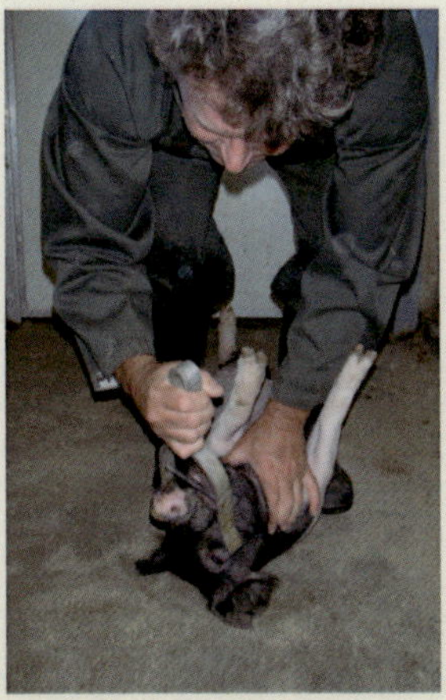

Figure 35. Examine the pig's mouth using a mouth gag.

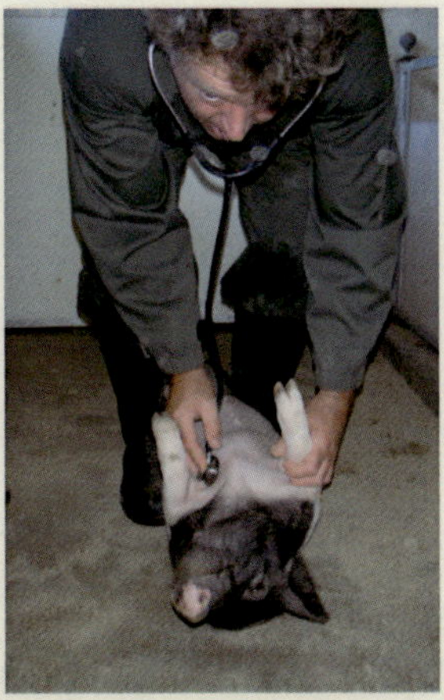

Figure 36. Auscultate heart and chest.

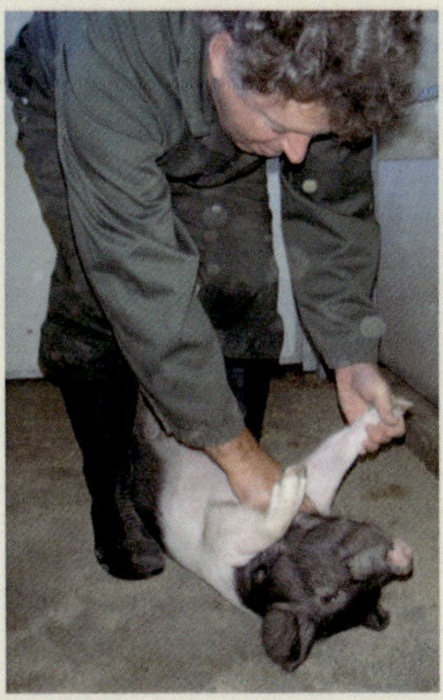

Figure 37. Examine left and right forelegs.

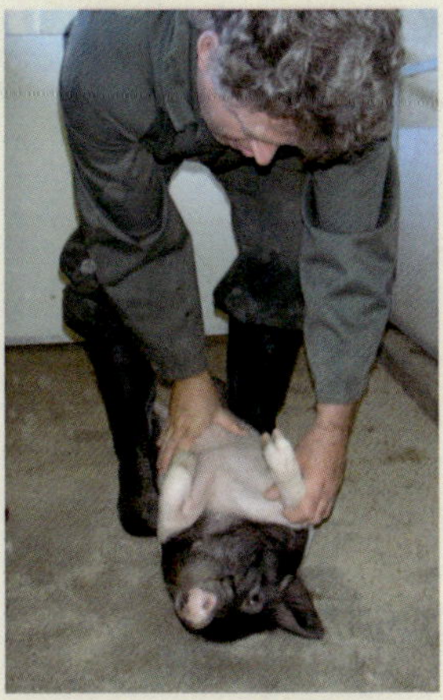

Figure 38. Examine the cranial ventral body wall.

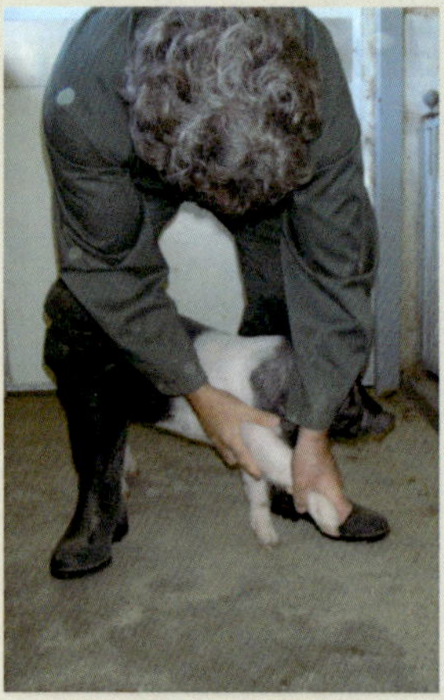

Figure 39. Relax your left foot from the shoulder and the pig will rotate onto its feet.

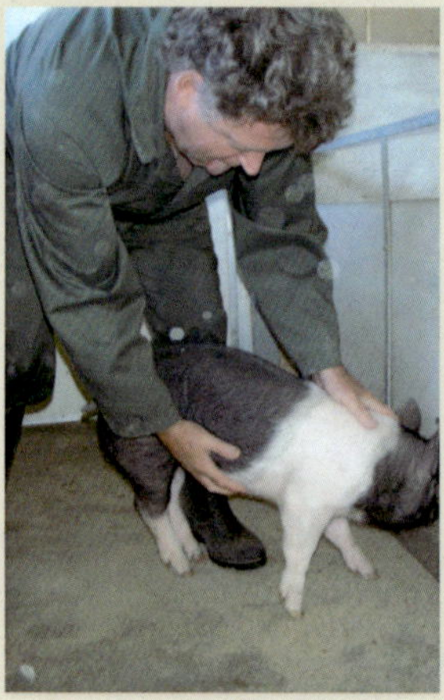

Figure 40. Examine the dorsal body wall as the pig moves away.

2

NORMAL BEHAVIOUR IN PIGS

THE BASICS

The basis of animal welfare revolves around the five "freedoms":

1. Freedom from thirst, hunger or malnutrition.
2. Freedom from thermal or physical discomfort.
3. Freedom from pain, injury or disease.
4. Freedom from fear and distress.
5. Freedom to express a normal pattern of behaviour.

However, in order to recognise that an animal's welfare is being compromised, it is imperative that the clinician understands and appreciates the normal repertoire of pig behaviours and expectations.

BOAR BREEDING OR STUD BEHAVIOUR

POSITIVE BEHAVIOURAL SIGNS

- Emptying of the prepuce on entry.
- Urinating looking at the collection stool.
- Salivating and chomping at collection stool.
- Smelling the collection stool.
- Chatting to the collection stool.
- Nudging of the collection stool.
- Barking/grunting at the collection stool.
- Rubbing the underline of the collection stool.
- Mounting and re-mounting the collection stool.
- Thrusting upon mounting the collection stool.
- Extension of penis upon mounting the collection stool.
- Paddling while on the collection stool.

NEGATIVE BEHAVIOURAL SIGNS

- Shying away from the collection stool.
- Shying away from the stockperson.
- Looking at the stockperson while he/she handles the underline of the boar.
- Entering into sleeping/covered area when asked to leave the pen.
- Lying down in sleeping/covered area when asked to leave the pen.
- Lying down in the collection area.
- Running around boar pen in a disturbed manner.
- Failure to interact with the collection stool.
- Failure to interact with the stockperson.
- Dismounting at stockperson's attempts to handle the boar.
- Failure to achieve an erection.
- Failure to achieve a fully coordinated ejaculation response.

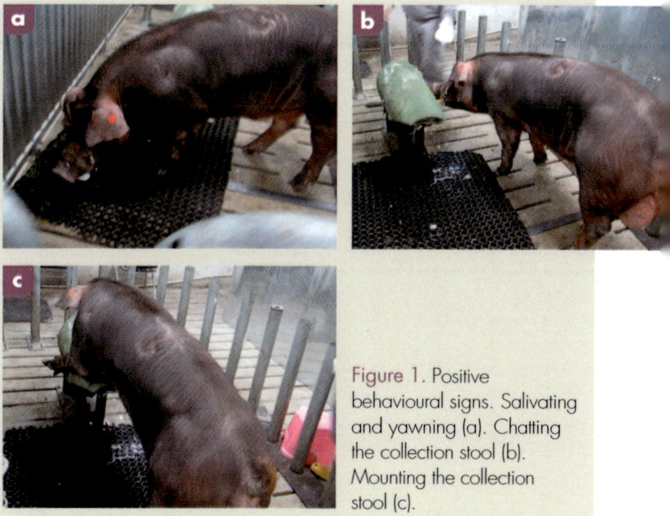

Figure 1. Positive behavioural signs. Salivating and yawning (a). Chatting the collection stool (b). Mounting the collection stool (c).

SOW BEHAVIOUR

THE SIGNS OF OESTRUS

PRO-OESTRUS

- In gilts, the vulva swells, but this is not consistent in the sow.
- The vulva becomes congested.
- The udder develops in gilts.
- The female becomes nervous and easily disturbed.
- She is ridden by other sows, but does not remain immobile.
- Vaginal wall becomes reddened (congested).
- Clitoris becomes more prominent.
- Vaginal fluid thickens, producing strands between fingers.

OESTRUS

- The vulva reddening starts to subside.
- There is a slight mucous vulval discharge.
- The female starts to mount other sows, and if mounted starts to stand.
- She emits a characteristic high-pitched grunt.
- She actively seeks boars.
- She has a decreased appetite.
- She 'stands' to back pressure, particularly in the presence of a boar.
- If a Large White, she pricks her ears.
- Stands with tail upright and flicking up and down.
- She has rub marks.
- She has a clean vulva in outdoor units (post service).
- She rubs and is attracted to stockpeople.
- Her eyes have glazed over.
- She allows coitus.

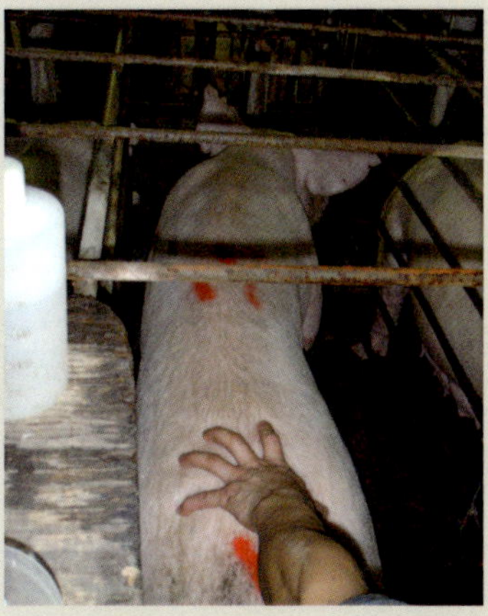

Figure 2. Stands to back pressure.

OESTRUS BEHAVIOUR PATTERNS

In a textbook example, the sow will gradually become immobile to the point A at which she does not move for several hours (Fig. 3). This behaviour would then gradually wane and the animal will start moving again.

Clearly, this does not happen in practice. Figure 3 describes a population of individual sows. It does not describe the events in a single individual.

Figure 3. Oestrus behaviour (population).

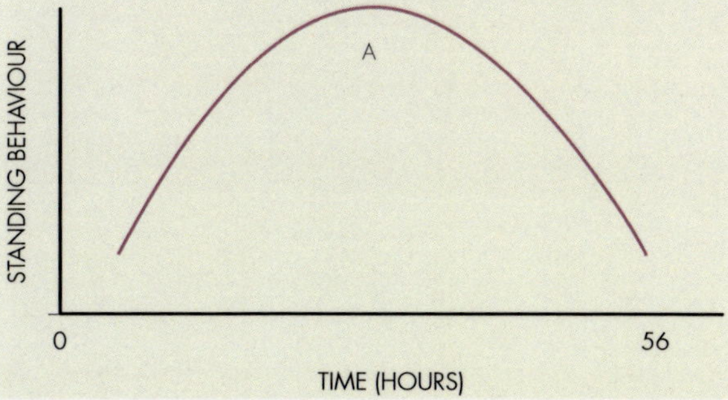

During oestrus, the individual sow becomes more and then less interested in the boar. The pattern of oestrus behaviour is better represented by Figure 4.

Figure 4. Oestrus behaviour (individual). The sow "switches in and out of oestrus".

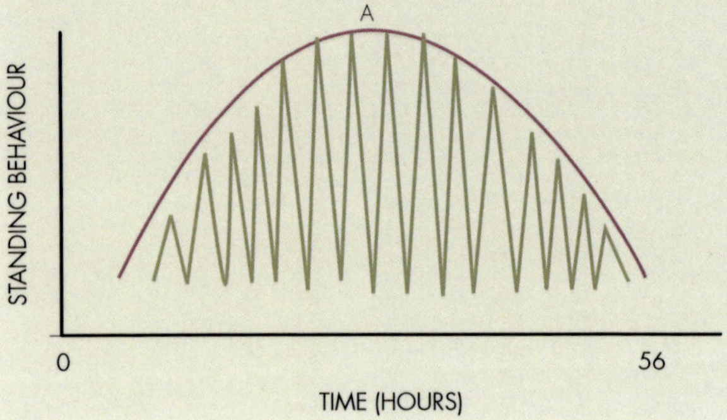

What happens around point A?

Let's examine the events around point A in some detail (Fig. 5). If we accept the following:

- The sow is in the middle of oestrus.
- The signs of oestrus wax and wane in intensity and the sow is not always responsive.
- All sows and boars are individuals.

The following questions can be asked:

- How long is the sow in heat i.e. time length B?
- How long is the sow not in heat i.e. time length C?

Figure 5. Oestrus behaviour around point A.

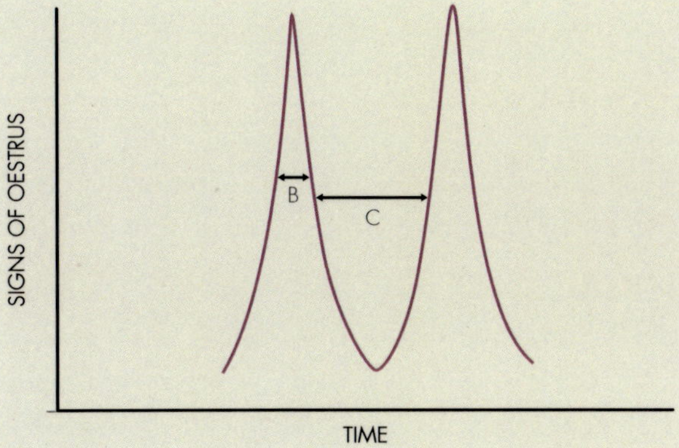

Research in this area is still limited; however, based on work in gilts and personal experiences regarding length B, the gilt is in heat for 10-15 minutes. This is when she will allow boars to mate with them. It is interesting to consider who initiates the end of mating. In many cases it is the sow who, by fidgeting and moving around, finishes mating with the boar sliding off.

Length C is more controversial and appears to be more variable. However, the gilt is not in heat for a time interval of 45 minutes. This interval partially depends on the degree of "satisfaction" the sow receives during mating. There is also a degree of submission in the presence of a keen boar.

FARROWING SIGNS AND BEHAVIOUR

Assuming farrowing at 115 days (with later litters this is increasing to 116-117days):

Time before/ after farrowing	Event	
-5 days	Foetal production of corticosteroids	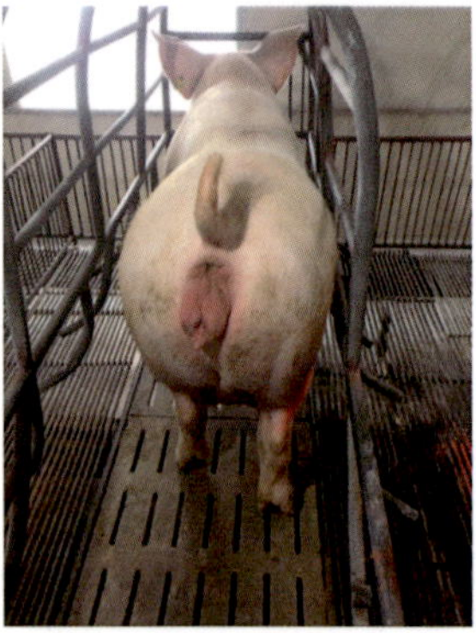
-4 days	• Progressive swelling of vulva. • Vulva becomes redder. • Mammary glands develop.	
-2 days	Individual mammary glands easily visible	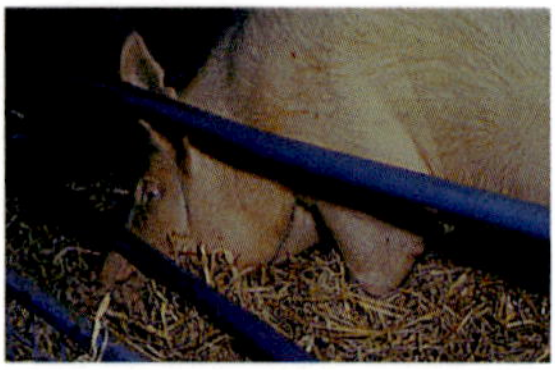
-1 day	Sow becomes restless	
	Nest making starts	
	Sow stops eating	
	Milk can be expressed from nipple	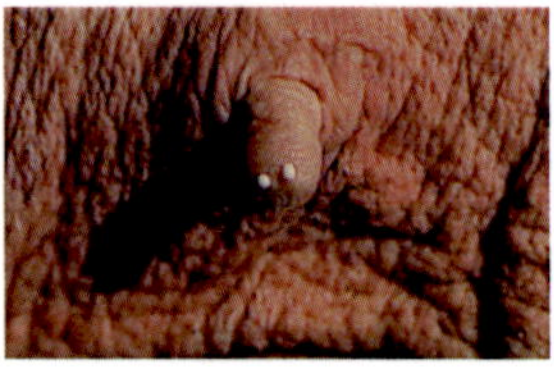
-12 hours	Sow lies down with periods of restlessness with clawing and chomping of bedding materials	
60-75% of sows farrow at night		

Time before/ after farrowing	Event	
-1 hour	Sow settles down in lateral recumbency	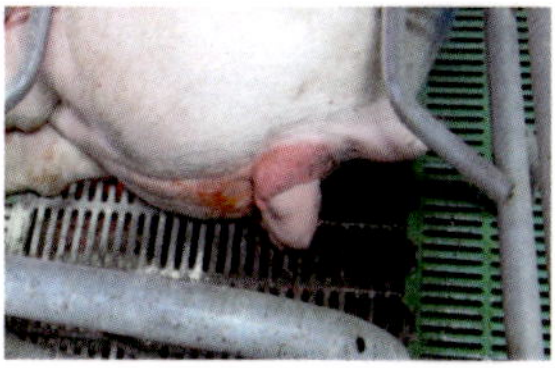
	Intermittent straining and paddling of legs	
-10 minutes	Passage of small quantity of foetal fluid	
	Marked twitching of tail	
	Pain and abdominal effort/straining	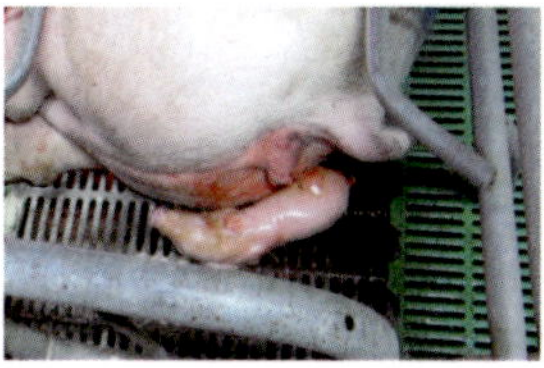
	Leg movement in time with contractions	
0	Passage of first piglet	
+ 0 to 3 hours	• Sow more relaxed • Passage of piglets every 10-20 minutes • Gilts may be restless after 2-3 piglets • Remaining piglets born within 3 hours	
	After last piglet: • Sow stands and urinates • Sow lies down quietly suckles	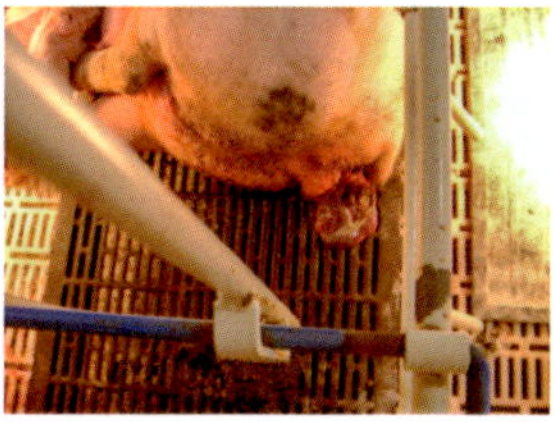
+ 4 to 8 hours	• Placental mass passed • The sow does little to assist her piglets • There is no sure way of knowing a sow has passed all her piglets and placenta. Watch sow behaviour for the next 24 hours	

PIGLET BEHAVIOUR

What attracts newborn piglets?

1. Vocalisation of sows.
2. Dark areas.
3. Afterbirth and birth fluids.
4. Movement along hair patterns.

NURSING PATTERNS AND CONSEQUENCES

Cyclic: sleeping and suckling (approximately once every hour).

Sow

- Slow grunting.
- Increase grunt rate.
- Rapid increase in grunt rate.
- Milk flow (15 sec).
- Grunting declines.
- Sleep or change position.

Piglet

- Assemble at udder.
- Nosing and teat location.
- Slow suckling.
- Rapid suckling.
- Slow suckling or nosing.
- Fall sleep.

TEAT ORDER

1. Established within 3 days.
2. Consistence often over 90%.
3. Less stable in large litters.
4. About 10% of piglets use more than one teat.
5. Multiple teats are more common in small litters.
6. Unused teats regress.
7. When sow turns over, so does the piglet teat order, it is teat specific.

THE FIRST FOUR DAYS POSTWEANING

It is essential to get the weaned pig rapidly adapted to its new existence postweaning.

Feeding space from weaning until day 3

Provide troughs of a sufficient length so that all the newly weaned pigs can eat at the same time. Calculate 10 cm per pig (5 cm per pig if the trough allows pigs to eat from both sides). Thus 20 weaned pigs should have 1 m of trough space (if double-sided access).

Feeding protocols

Day of weaning

1. Wean the pigs and allow 2 hours for the weaners to acclimatise to their new environment. Ideally make several drinkers leak so that the weaners are attracted to them. Drink nipples should not be elevated or require a step up. Turkey drinkers can be very useful.
2. After two hours, go into the weaner pen and call the weaners by voice. Tap on the feed bucket and pour the gruel into the trough, filling the whole length of the trough. The weaners will

rapidly come up to you and start swarming around you and the trough. Stay still and gently talk to the weaners. It is essential to provide an amount of food in the trough that the weaners will eat in 10 minutes. If the trough is emptied in less than 10 minutes, increase volume by 20 % at the next feed. Place dry creep feed in the normal feeders by hand.

3. Repeat step 2 twice, at 1.5 hour-intervals.

At the end of the first day of weaning, after the third feeding opportunity is finished, turn off the lights to encourage the weaners to sleep.

WEANERS NOT EATING

Note and mark all weaners who shy away from the trough and refuse to eat at the first two occasions.

At the 3rd time, pick up all the weaners who have refused to eat. Place the weaner by the feed trough and encourage the weaner to eat, using fingers if necessary.

Second day of weaning

- Feed gruel to the pigs every two hours. Feed six times today.
- Note the increases in volume and dryness of the feed.
- At the end of the day, switch off the lights and allow the pigs to sleep.
- The short feeding interval aims to prevent the weaners from screaming after their lost mothers.
- Increase the amount of feed in the normal feeders, still feed by hand.

Third day of weaning

- Continue feeding gruel and extend the feeding interval to every three hours, i.e. four feeding times.
- Turn on normal creep feeders.

Fourth day of weaning

- Feed only a single gruel feed, two hours after daybreak. Observe the weaners' behaviour.
- If the pigs are well settled, no further hand feeding is required.
- Ensure normal feeders are working and adjusted as required.
- If everything is working well, provide one single meal and just water to make the weaners realise the gruel feeding is over.

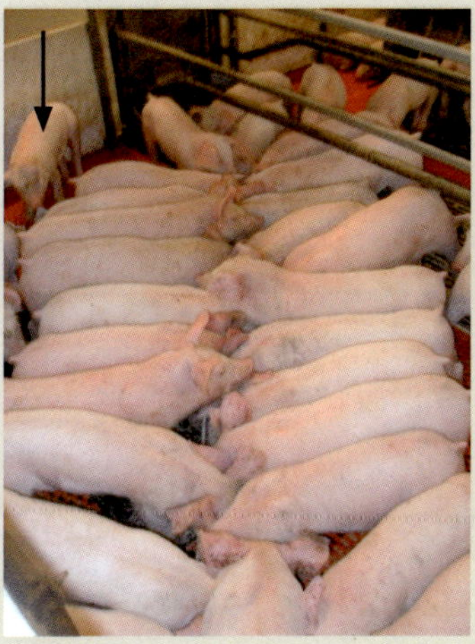

Figure 6. Weaners eating out of a trough feeder. Be concerned about the isolated pig (arrow).

CARING FOR THE LOWER-ORDER PIGS

If the 'bottom' 10 % of pigs at weaning is placed into a separate environment, it is possible to modify their gruel-feeding programme to last 7 days, rather than the 3 days described.

Whatever you do, it is essential to get the pigs eating normal creep feed as soon as possible, otherwise a "double weaning" event will occur, which will set the pigs back significantly.

COMFORT ASSESSMENT

INSTANT ASSESSMENT. THE LYING PATTERN

Too cold

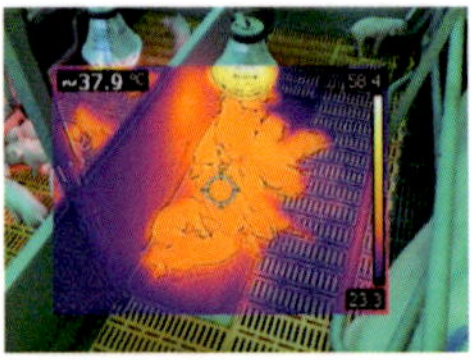

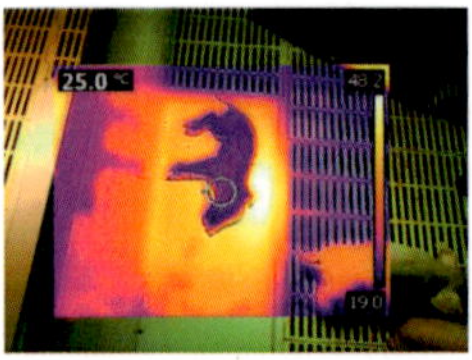

- Lies on the floor with its legs tucked under its body to reduce floor contact. Lies huddled with other pigs. Lies close to a wall.
- Pigs may shiver and may become hairy.
- Larger pigs seem unable to adopt this tucked-under position for very long and tend to lie semi-recumbent with their legs tucked towards their body.
- The infrared camera is a great tool to assist examination of the lying pattern. The first picture shows a failure of the heat mat and the piglets are then piling under the light to keep warm. The second one shows a hypothermic piglet (blue on infrared)

Comfortable

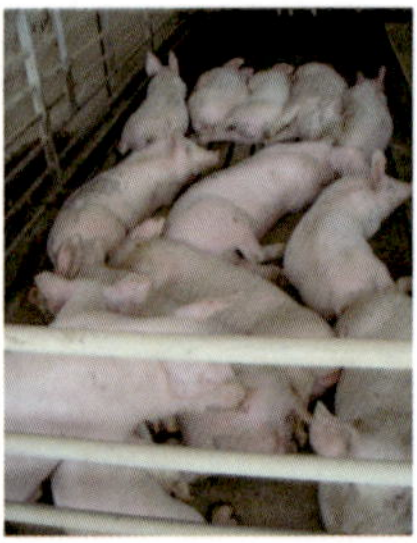

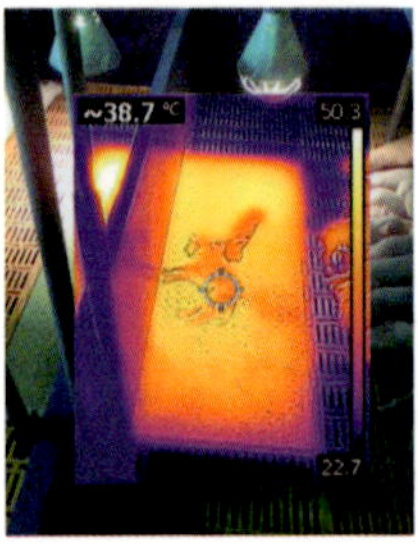

Within a group of pigs there will be a variety of lying patterns. The main group of pigs will sleep together in a pile, while other pigs will be lying spread out but with maximum floor contact. These separated pigs will be the more dominant pigs. The lower-order pigs will lie on the edge of the main group. Pigs sleep with legs stretched out from the body. With the infrared camera the heat mat should be the same temperature as the pig, so the pig does not loose heat to the floor.

Too hot

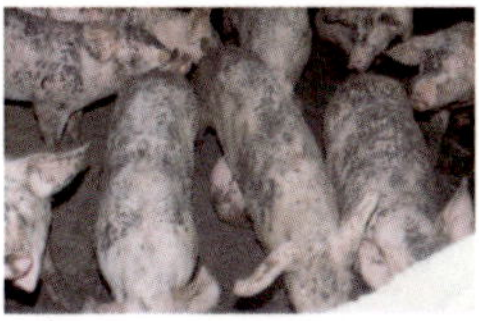

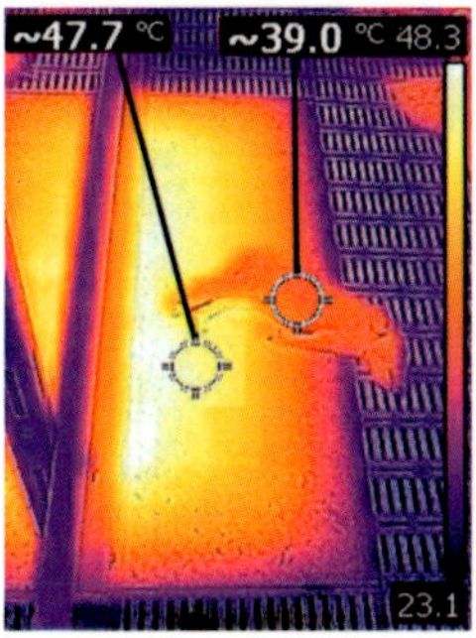

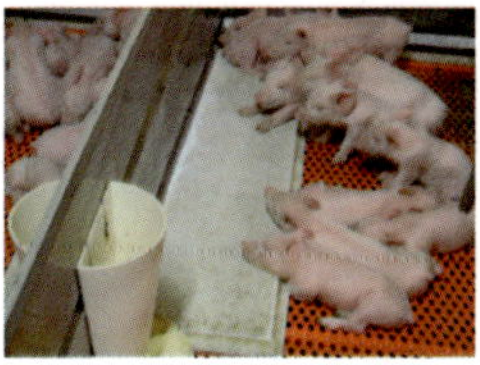

- Pigs are panting (respiration rate > 40 per minute).
- Pigs are generally dirty.
- Lie away from other pigs, sometimes against a cold wall.
- They do not pile.
- Lie in any wet/cooler area.
- They will dig into earth/bedded floors.
- They will avoid the hot area, placing only head or feet into hot area.

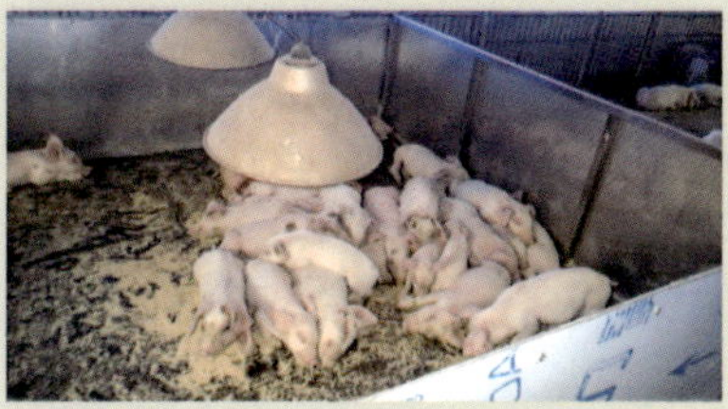

Figure 7. Chilled piglets will huddle and pile up.

LONG-TERM ASSESSMENT. DEFECATION BEHAVIOUR

Pigs are inherently clean animals and avoid lying in faeces. From a few days of age pigs, will become toilet trained and only defecate in a specific area of the environment.

The pig's need for a toilet area is very similar to our own.

Compare and contrast the needs for a defecation area and a sleeping area. Are the farm's pens designed to accommodate both?

Defecation area	Sleeping area
Wet	Dry
Cold	Warm/hot
Draughty	No draughts
Dark	Light
Private	Open
Uncomfortable	Comfortable

It is possible to assist the pig determine their defecation area.

- Prepare the house with the above considerations in mind.
- Help the pig choose by preparing a defecation area.
- Help the pig choose by preparing a sleeping area.

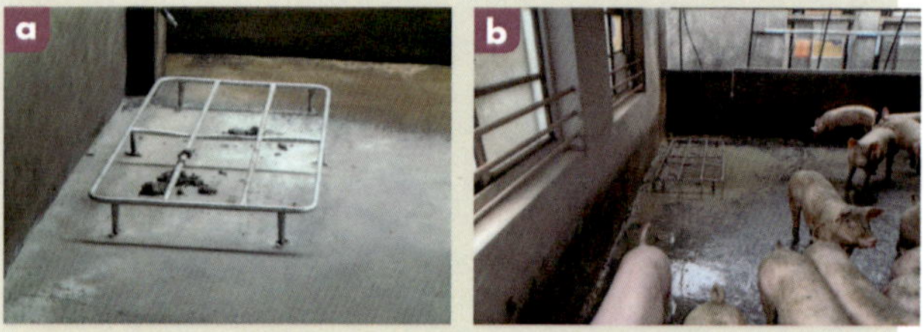

Figure 8. Room preparation with faeces from the same group placed in the defecation area (a). The defecation area in use (b).

PIGS AT PLAY

Any stockperson watching a group of pigs will soon be amused to observe their play activities. Play prepares them for situations and trains survival skills.

Pigs are extremely intelligent animals with a degree of complex behaviours that match if not surpass that of domestic dogs. Unlike cattle and sheep, pigs exhibit greater inquisitive and individualist behavioural patterns. This is obvious to anyone who tries moving a group of pigs. In many ways, pigs are more like people than we would like to admit.

Providing an environment where pigs can explore their play behaviour can help relieve stress and allow the pig to better cope if their environment is temporarily adverse.

COMPANY

Pigs will gain comfort and support from other pigs and other animals. Pigs should not be kept in isolation. There may be obvious exceptions, e.g. if the pig is under treatment for meningitis or severe lameness (Fig. 9).

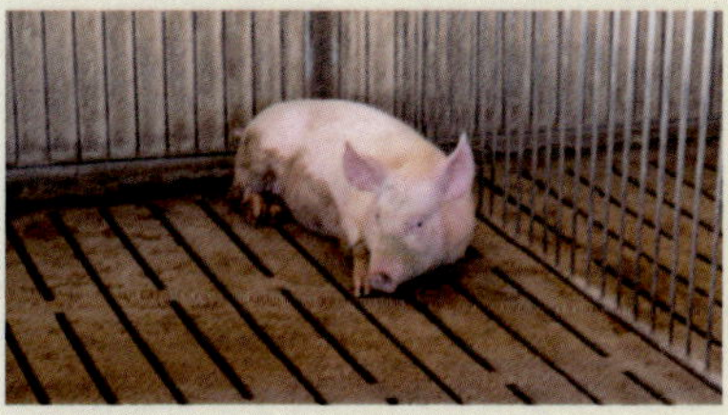

Figure 9. Pig kept in isolation.

ENVIRONMENTAL ENRICHMENT

Adult pigs

Adult pigs generally have a lower requirement to play with items placed in their pen. However, playing music to adult sows can have a calming effect (Fig. 10).

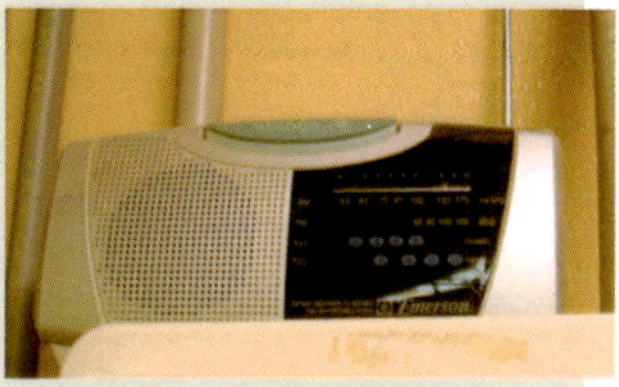

Figure 10. Music can have a calming effect.

Farrowing sows can be provided with chopped paper, straw and hay to allow them to act out their nest-building behaviour (Fig. 11).

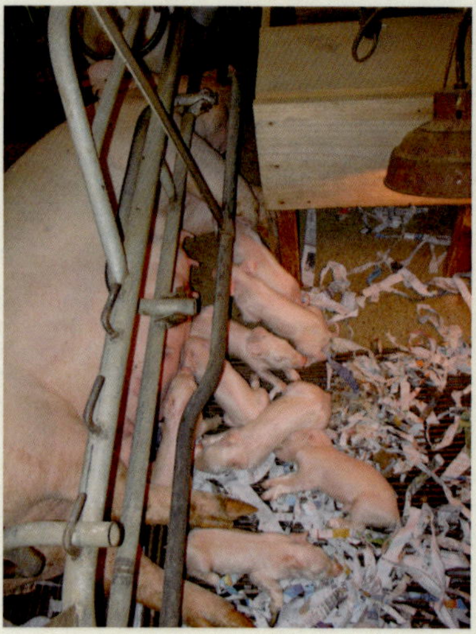

Figure 11. Chopped paper, straw and hay to allow sows express their nesting behaviour.

Wean-to-finish pigs

All wean-to-finish pigs should be provided with toys within the pen.

The simplest toys are often the most effective. Pigs love to play with chains, rattles, large plastic bottles, rubber belting, old boots and feedbags (Fig. 12).

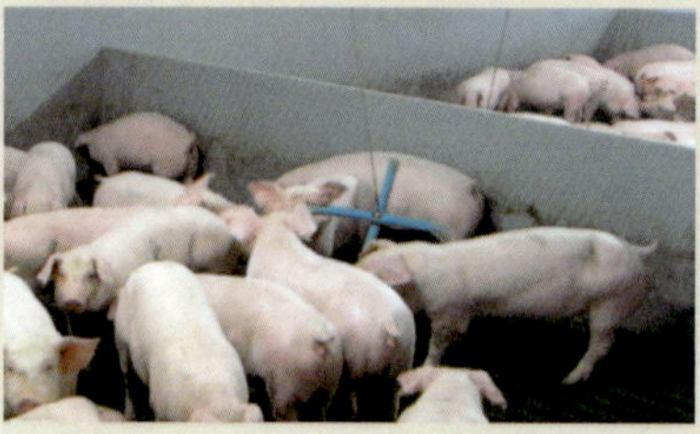

Figure 12. Pigs love to play with simple toys.

HANDLING AND MOVING PIGS

Most pigs are not used to being handled. They become very vocal when caught and will not settle easily. Pigs will work as a herd or as individuals. Before moving a group of pigs, think of escape routes you would take and then try to block them.

PIG: FIELD OF VIEW

Pigs will generally try and face their handler, as they are more vulnerable if approached from behind. The stockperson should avoid the pig's blind spot and stand at an angle of about 60° behind the head, where, when moving forward, the pig will move forward as well.

Figure 13. Vision zones of pigs.

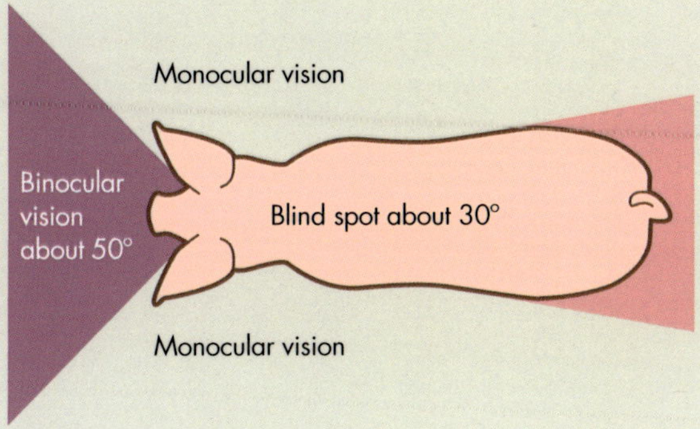

LOADING AREA DESIGN

Any pig to be transported must be fit to load onto the truck and unload at the arrival point.

Moving pigs

- Pigs can be moved by a stockman's voice; hands and gestures; boards; flags or paddles.
- The pigs should not be hit by any of these moving aids.
- Electric prodders should not be used to move pigs.
- Pigs move easier if the stockperson has fully planned the move.

Basic design

- The loading area should have no sharp turns.
- The loading area should be free of any protrusions, such as nails or bolts.
- There should be no steps or gaps in the walkway.
- Ideally there should be no slope to the loading area.
- If a slope is necessary, it should be 20° at the most.
- The ramp for finishing pigs should be 0.9-1.0 m wide, sufficient for two 120 kg pigs.
- Have a see-through fence down the middle of the ramp, so the pigs can see each other.
- The ramp sides should be solid at 1.0 m high.
- The loading area should be well lit (250 lux).
- Avoid any sharp contrast between dark and light. This includes wet patches.
- The loading area should protect the pigs and staff from the weather (heat and cold).
- The ramp should have a walkway for staff.
- There should be a flat area of 2 meters long at the top of the ramp.
- A biosecurity creep bar should be placed at the top of the ramp.
- Do not allow the farm staff to enter the truck.
- Do not allow the truck driver to enter the ramp area.
- Cleats in the ramp should be 2.5 cm metal rods separated by a gap more than the pig's feet but not wide enough to allow the pig to slip.

Figure 14. Plan of loading area.

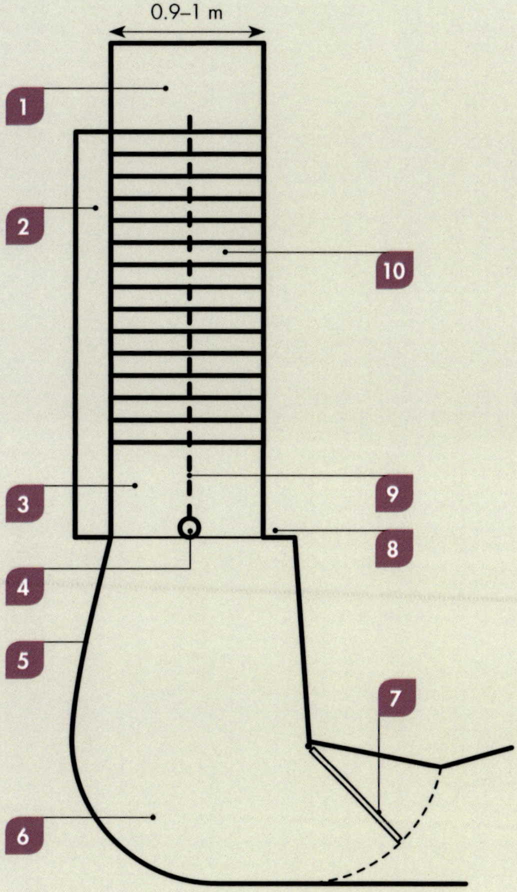

1. Level dock (1 sq m)
2. Stockperson walkway
3. Level area (1 sq m)
4. Entrance restrictor
5. Wall (2 m)
6. Round corner
7. Gate
8. Offset step
9. See through fence
10. Raiseable ramp (<20 degrees)

Figure 15. Illustration of loading area.

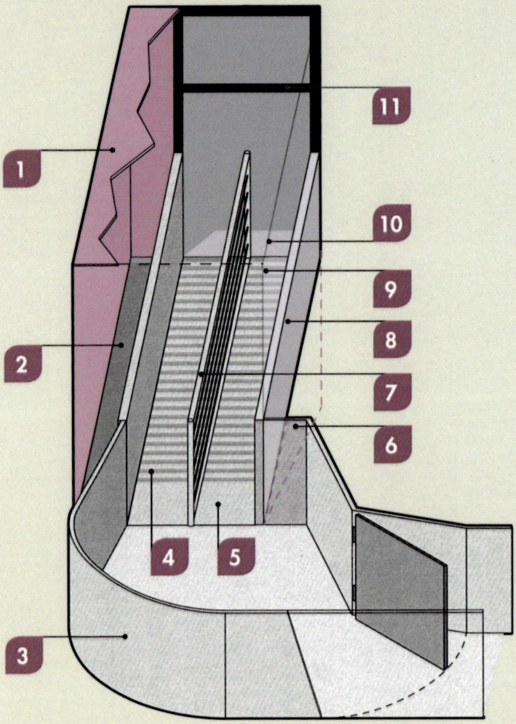

1. Cover protecting staff and pigs
2. Stockperson walkway
3. Sidewall (slight angle)
4. Cleats (2.5 cm, round metal)
5. Level area
6. Offset step
7. See through fence
8. Solid side 1 m
9. Raiseable ramp (<20 degrees)
10. Level area before truck
11. Biosecurity creep bar

3

DISORDERS OF THE PIG ACCORDING TO CLINICAL SIGNS

ABORTION

There is a wide range of possible causes of abortion in the pig. The majority of abortions are non-infectious and some 90 % cannot be linked to a specific cause. Around 1.5 % of all services fail to farrow due to abortion. Abortion can occur at any time of pregnancy after day 11 until day 112. However, the loss of embryos around day 20 without the loss of the corpora lutea will not result in abortion; the sow will enter a period of pseudopregnancy and recycle after day 63 postmating.

NON-INFECTIOUS CAUSES

Seasonal effects

70 % of all abortions fall into this category. In nature, it is normal for sows to farrow in the spring, and therefore, there is a natural tendency for pregnancies to be lost in summer and autumn. Many factors may be involved in the summer infertility/autumn abortion syndrome, such as variable daily temperatures, reduction in light length, effect of heat, loss of appetite in the summer. Ensure your breeding targets accommodate any seasonal impact. Even production is essential.

Environmental abortions

Sows may be subjected to stress factors relating to their environment: draughts, excessive heat stress, inadequate cooling, change in feeding routines, changes in stockpeople, bullying when introduced into a new group and trauma from moving through narrow doorways. All of these factors, alone or in combination can result in abortion in the individual sow. Injections can also result in abortions, particularly associated with some vaccines.

Mycotoxins

Mycotoxin	Source	Toxic threshold	Effect
Aflatoxin	• *Aspergillus flavus* • *Aspergillus parasiticus*	>0.2 ppm	• Hepatitis • Stunted growth • Reduced feed intake • Immunosuppression
Deoxynivalenol (DON), aka Vomitoxin	*Fusarium* spp.	>0.5 ppm	Reduced feed intake
Ergot	*Claviceps purpurea*	>1000 ppm	• Reduced feed intake • Agalactia • Gangrene
Fumonisins	• *Fusarium moniliforme* • *Fusarium proliferatum*	>25 ppm	• Liver dysfunction • Pulmonary oedema
Ochratoxin, citrinin	• *Aspergillus ochraceus* • *Penicillium viridicatum* • *Penicillium citrinum*	>0.2 ppm	• Renal lesions • Immunosuppression
T-2 toxin, DAS (trichotecenes)	*Fusarium* spp.	>3 ppm	• Reduced feed intake • Immunosuppression
Zearalenone	*Fusarium graminearum*	>1 ppm	• Infertility, anoestrus • Pseudopregnancy • Enlarged vulva in weaners
Gossypol (plant toxin)	Cottonseed	>200 ppm	Reduced feed intake

Note: 1 ppm = 1 mg/kg; 1 ppb = 0.001 mg/kg or 1 µg/kg

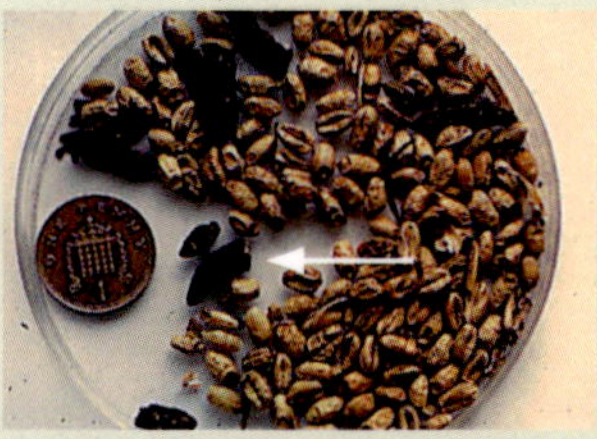

Figure 1. Ergot (arrow).

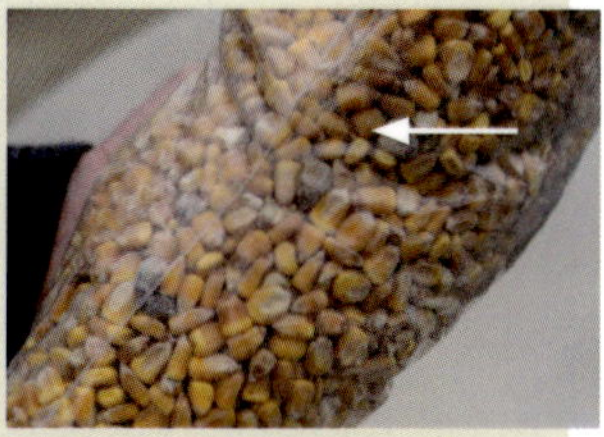

Figure 2. *Fusarium* on maize – Zearalenone 10 ppm.

INFECTIOUS CAUSES

There are many infectious causes of abortion. Pathogens can cause abortion through one of two major routes:

a. Luteolysis (luteal regression). High body temperatures will cause the release of endogenous prostaglandins, which induce luteolysis, causing the termination of pregnancy. Examples include swine influenza, erysipelas or African and Classical swine fever.

b. Death of the piglet/placentitis. Diseases that kill piglets include brucellosis, the porcine reproductive and respiratory syndrome (PRRS), Aujeszky's disease, Japanese encephalitis.

Brucellosis

Causal agent		*Brucella suis* bacterium biovars 1, 2 and 3.
Age group		All ages can be affected. Clinical signs are rare.
Clinical signs	Sows	Abortion, infertility and severe metritis.
	Boars	Orchitis (infection of testes) and infertility (Fig. 3).
	Piglets, weaners	Posterior paralysis and lameness.
Other remarks		Brucellosis has a zoonotic potential.

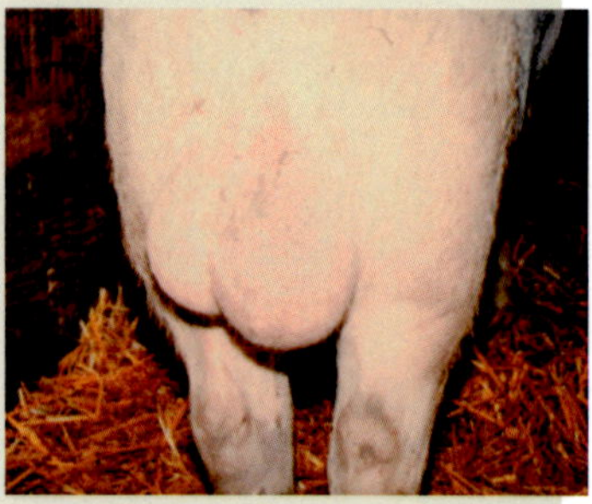

Figure 3. A boar with orchitis due to *Brucella suis*.

Leptospirosis

Causal agent		Leptospira are corkscrew-shaped bacteria (spirochaetes) present in all parts of the world. There are five serovars that are important in pigs: *L. interrogans* serovar Pomona (most important), Australis (Bratislava), Tarassovi, Canicola, Icterohaemorrhagiae and Grippotyphosa.
Age group		Any age group, but mainly adults.
Clinical signs	Acute	• As signs are very nonspecific and only affect individuals, this infection is often missed. • Anorexia, pyrexia and listlessness. • With *L. icterohaemorrhagiae*, the animals can be very ill and jaundiced (Fig. 4), and weaners are also affected. Check water line for a dead rat.
	Chronic	Abortions, stillbirths, weak piglets and other vague reproductive signs.
Postmortem lesions	Acute	Postmortem findings can be very limited in acute cases.
	Chronic	Kidneys: scattered small grey foci of a focal interstitial nephritis (Fig. 5). However, many other diseases can cause similar findings while *Leptospira* can also be isolated from kidneys without pathological lesions.
Other remarks		*Leptospira* are zoonotic pathogens.

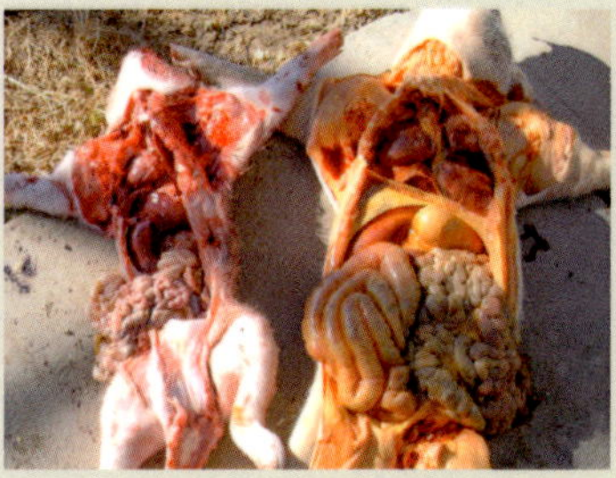

Figure 4. Normal and jaundiced pig (yellow).

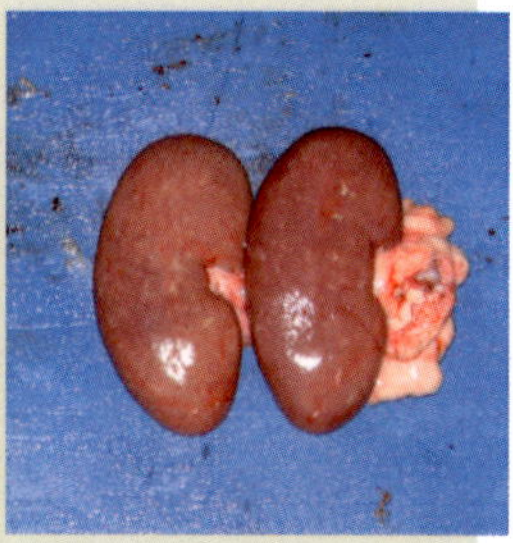

Figure 5. Interstitial nephritis, commonly associated with *L. pomona*.

Porcine reproductive and respiratory syndrome (PRRS)

Causal agent		Porcine reproductive and respiratory syndrome virus (enveloped RNA virus). A typical outbreak on a naive farrow to finish farm is an abortion storm with many pigs off their food.
Age group		All ages: • Adult sows (reproductive signs, mild fever and anorexia). • Piglets through to finishing (secondary infections).
Clinical signs	Naive herds	• Reproductive losses and a decreased farrowing rate. • Early farrowings, at 105 to 112 days. • Increase in stillborn, mummified and weak live-born pigs. • Increased preweaning mortality, often associated with an increase in bacterial infections (diarrhoea, greasy pig disease). • Increased numbers of unthrifty pigs post weaning. • Increased nursery mortality often associated with an increase in bacterial infections (postweaning diarrhoea and meningitis).
	Established herds	**Neonatal piglets** • Respiratory distress, unthrifty pigs. • Increased secondary bacterial infections such as diarrhoea (scour) and pneumonia.
		Growing pigs • Increased mortality, decreased appetite, fever, rough hair coat, unthrifty pigs. • Increased respiratory problems, pneumonia and atrophic rhinitis. • Increased secondary bacterial infections (meningitis, greasy pig disease) (Fig. 6).
		Adult pigs Can cause major reproductive problems with massive abortions ("abortion storms") (Fig. 7). In combination with other pathogens, a highly pathogenic type 2 variant in China has been associated with high mortality and unique lesions throughout the body.

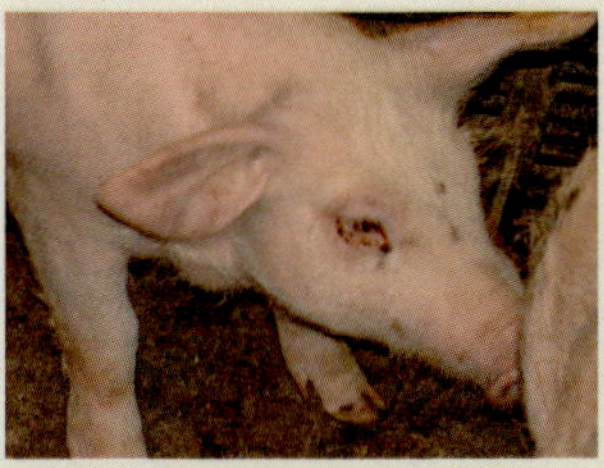

Figure 6. Pig with conjunctivitis due to underlying PRRSV infection.

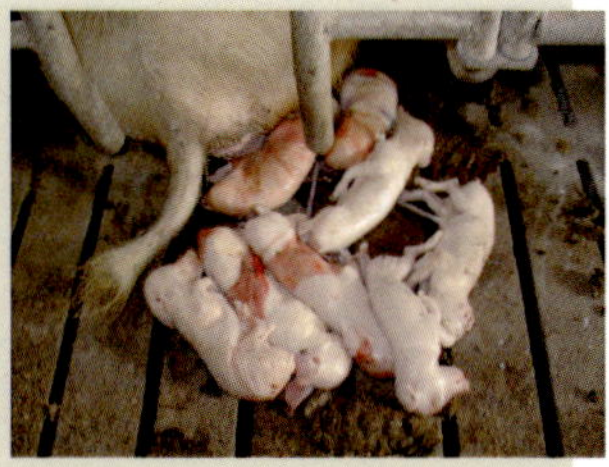

Figure 7. Abortions.

COUGHING PIGS IN THE FINISHING HERD

ENZOOTIC PNEUMONIA (EP) / *MYCOPLASMA* PNEUMONIA. PORCINE RESPIRATORY DISEASE COMPLEX (PRDC)

Causal agent	*Mycoplasma hyopneumoniae*. A mycoplasma is a kind of bacterium without a cell wall. These organisms will not react to penicillin antibiotics. Enzootic pneumonia may not require *M. hyopneumoniae*, although this agent is often involved.
Age group	Common in growing and finishing pigs.
Involved factors	**Complicating factors** • Bacteria: There are a number of bacteria and mycoplasmas that can infect the lower respiratory tract, often as a secondary infection. These include *Pasteurella*, *Streptococcus* and *Actinobacillus pleuropneumoniae* (APP). *Haemophilus parasuis* (Glässer's disease) also plays a contributing role in postweaning respiratory disease. • Viruses: These include PRRSV, swine influenza, porcine circovirus type 2 and porcine respiratory coronavirus (PRCV). Aujeszky's disease (pseudorabies) virus may play a pivotal role. • Parasites (*Ascaris*, lungworm) may also play a role. **Environmental factors** Many factors for which the stockperson is responsible: • Air: Excessive 24 hour temperature variations. Draughts. High ammonia levels. • Floor: Overstocking, rough floors. • Water: Poor water flow. Insufficient number of drinking nipples. • Feed: Dusty feed. Poor feed availability.

Clinical signs	• Coughing, laboured breathing. • Fever may be present (temperatures of 40.5 to 41 °C imply a complicated enzootic pneumonia). • Variable growth rates, unthrifty appearance, reduced appetite and increased postweaning mortality. • In naive herds, sows may abort and die.
Other remarks	*Mycoplasma hyopneumoniae* destroy the cilial cells lining the trachea and bronchi (upper airways), which act as an escalator that help to protect the lung from dust and disease particles. With the cilia destroyed, pathogens can enter the lungs with ease, causing areas to collapse (Fig. 8) and the pig progressively becomes short of air. The collapsed areas become infected with other pathogens and the pig finally succumbs to the disease load.

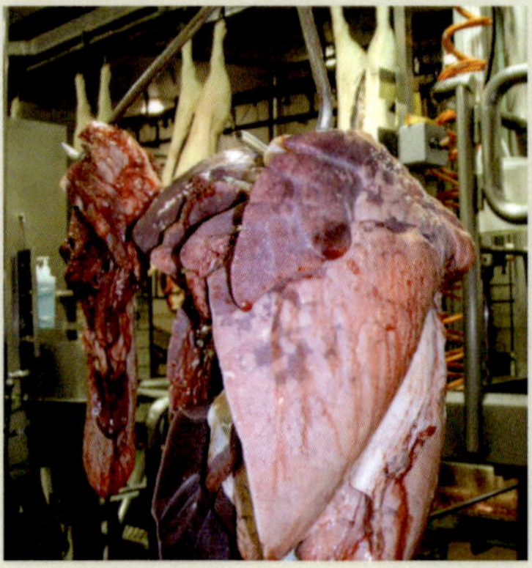

Figure 8. The diseased (collapsed) areas are darker than the normal, light parts of the lung.

SWINE INFLUENZA

Causal agent	Swine influenza virus, which belongs to the Influenza type A virus group: • H_1N_1, H_3N_2 and reassortant H_1N_2 are problematic. H_1N_1 with avian and human internal genes has been observed. • There are 16 H and 9 N types providing a lot of potential. There are currently at least seven different pig-adapted influenza viruses.
Age group	All ages can be affected.

Clinical signs	**Naive herds** Explosive outbreaks with all or many animals becoming ill at the same time. The disease is much more common in spring and autumn. • Inactivity, depression, huddling/piling. • Anorexia. • Breathing is laboured, often with an open mouth. If the animals are moved, many cough, some uncontrollably (paroxysmal coughing). • Nasal discharge, puffy eyes. • The rectal temperature can reach 40.5–41.5 °C. In breeding stock, this can result in abortions, infertility (a boar can become sub-fertile for 6 weeks), production of small, weak litters and increased stillbirths. • Weight loss may be seen as the disease progresses. • Mortality is generally low. • Recovery generally starts 5 to 7 days after the first clinical signs.
	Established herds • Annual reinfection, possibly from carrier pigs or the natural spread to younger naive pigs who present few signs in the summer months. • Reduced water (-10%). Monitoring water use may be helpful to predict an outbreak.
Other remarks	Swine influenza may have a zoonotic potential.

DEAD PIGS AROUND THE FARM

The main causes are: abdominal catastrophe, gastric ulcer, classical swine fever (hog cholera) or African swine fever.

- If sudden death in individual pigs is seen in the nursery, mulberry heart disease is a likely cause.
- If there are dead pigs in the growing/finishing barn, APP is likely.
- If a sow is suddenly found dead in the breeding barn, cystitis and pyelonephritis should be considered.

ABDOMINAL CATASTROPHE

A cause of sudden death in adults is an abdominal catastrophe, characterised by a torsion/twist (figs. 9 and 10) or rupture of the abdominal organs (fig. 11). The intestinal tract is twisted at the mesentery root or is associated with a mesenteric tear (fig. 12). Occasionally, the spleen or a liver lobe can become involved (fig. 13).

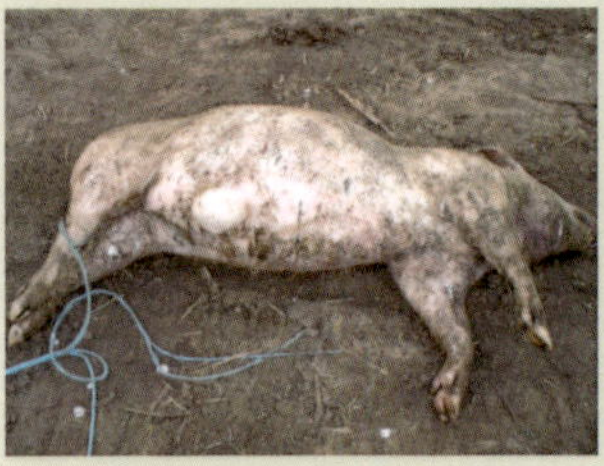

Figure 9. A pig that died due to an abdominal twist. The abdomen may be more bloated.

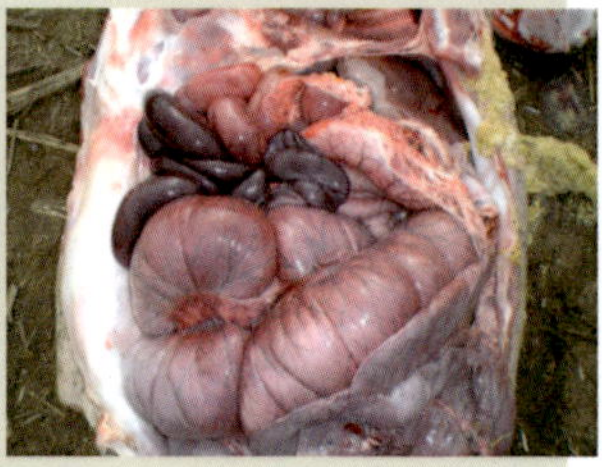

Figure 10. Gross postmortem view of the pig in Fig. 9, showing the intestinal torsion.

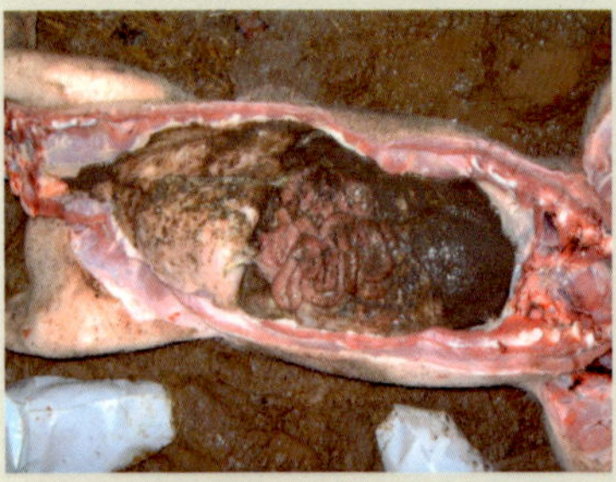

Figure 11. Rupture of the intestinal tract and release of intestinal contents into the abdomen.

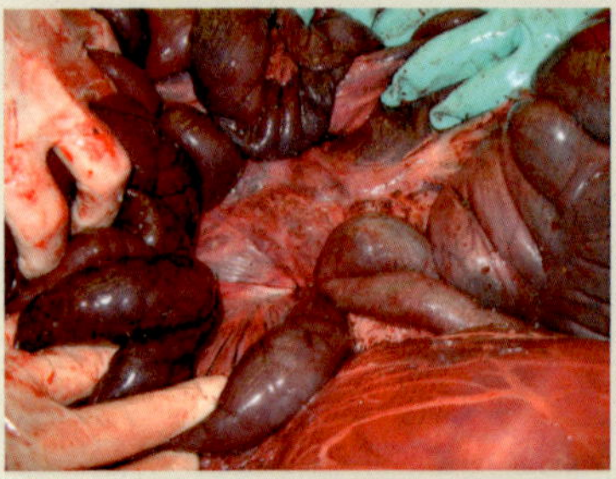

Figure 12. A twist at the root of the mesentery, the membrane that attaches the intestines to the abdominal wall.

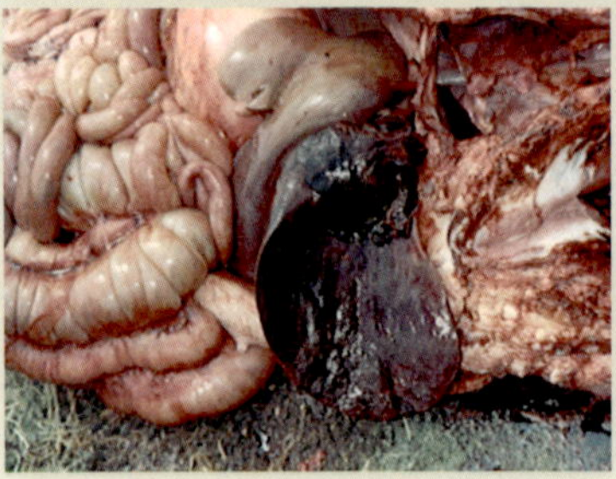

Figure 13. Torsion of a liver lobe, appearance in the abdomen and the liver laid out.

GASTRIC ULCERATION

Causes		Caused by not eating. The ulcer is aggravated by many factors including nutritional factors, stress and pathogens.
Age group		Any age group. More common in lactating sows and in grower pigs older than 8 weeks. The condition can occur in up to 100 % of groups of pigs, and rates of 50 % of sows and 60 % of growers.
Clinical signs	Peracute	• Death or collapse of apparently healthy animals. The animal may be pale (anaemic). • Acute death is associated when the ulcer invades an underlying large blood vessel.
	Acute	• Animals weak and wobbly on their legs. • Anaemic (pale) with an increased respiration rate. • Pain, causing pigs to grind their teeth and swish their tail in pain. • Animals lie down and fidget trying to find a comfortable position. • Bloody, tarry faeces (melaena). Note: in-feed copper also makes pigs' faeces dark. • Vomiting may be noted. • Anorexia (no appetite). The rectal temperature is normal. Subnormal temperatures generally indicate a poor prognosis.
	Chronic	• Same as acute clinical signs with weaker animals. This may be misdiagnosed as pneumonia in growers. • Sometimes, oesophageal entrance becomes narrow and a stricture occurs, causing the pigs to vomit shortly after feeding then run off rapidly. • Sometimes gastric ulceration is an incidental postmortem finding.
Postmortem lesions		• Peracute/acute cases: the stomach is filled with dark/black blood or a large blood clot (Fig. 14). The ulcer often has invaded an underlying large blood vessel. • In the more chronic cases: black streaks in the stomach contents. The large intestine is full of black tarry faeces (Fig. 15). • The ulcer can vary from a mild erosion to a large ulcer with a thickened, scarred wall boundary. Chronic ulcers may bleed more easily than the acute-looking ulcer due to the oozing of blood over a long period of time. • Stricture at the oesophageal entrance (Fig. 16).

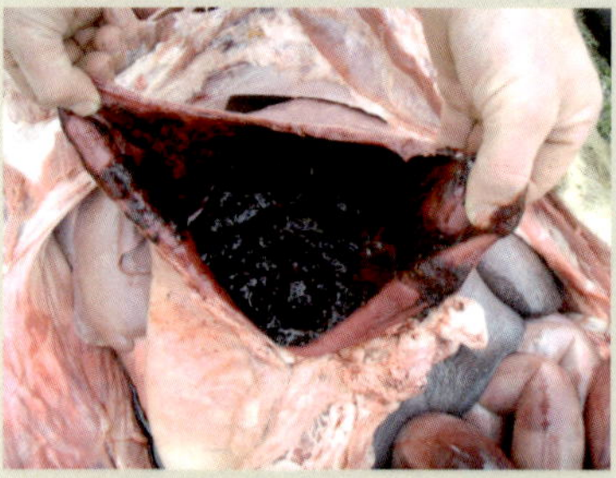

Figure 14. Haemorrhagic gastric ulcer and a stomach full of blood.

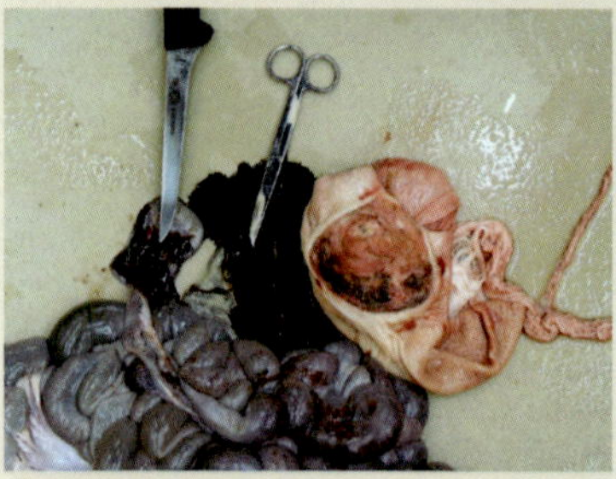

Figure 15. Gastric ulcer in a weaner.

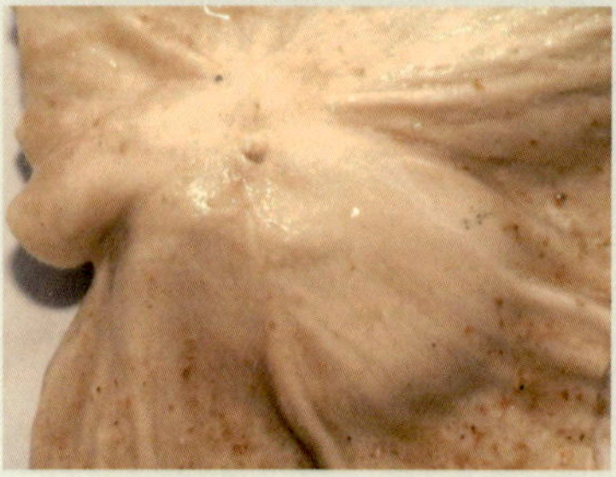

Figure 16. Chronic ulcer with scarring of the oesophageal entrance.

THE SWINE FEVERS – AFRICAN AND CLASSICAL SWINE FEVER (HOG CHOLERA)

Causal agent	**Classical swine fever (CSF)**: a *Flaviviridae* virus, genus *Pestivirus*. Enveloped RNA virus. **African swine fever (ASF):** enveloped DNA virus related to Poxviruses. Clinically, it is not possible to distinguish between CSF and ASF.
Age group	All age groups.

Clinical signs	Naive herds	• Initially, a few pigs appear drowsy and less active, with some anorexia.. • Within days, pigs will present with a marked fever (41–42 °C), with a reddening of the skin. • The pigs develop conjunctivitis and constipation leading to yellowish diarrhoea. • The pigs appear chilled and will huddle together. • A few pigs may convulse before they die. • Pigs start to die with a spreading purple discoloration of the skin. Death often occurs some 10 to 20 days postinfection. • In the adult herd, reproductive signs are seen: mass abortions. • Pigs that survive will be chronically affected with severe retardation of growth and often present with arched backs.
	Established herds	**Congenital infection** • Infection during pregnancy can result in abortion (Fig. 17), mummification, malformations (e.g. congenital tremor with cerebellar hypoplasia due to CSF infection), stillbirths and weak born piglets. • Piglets born from CSF-infected mothers may remain healthy but continually spread the disease throughout their lives.
		Rest of the herd In the rest of the herd, the infection may be inapparent. Chronically infected herds can be very difficult to identify.
Postmortem lesions	Peracute	The pigs may die so rapidly that there are few postmortem signs.
	Acute	• Multiple haemorrhages throughout the carcase (Fig. 18). • Swollen, oedematous and haemorrhagic lymph nodes. • The spleen will have large areas where the blood supply has been cut off (infarction), resulting in blood-filled blebs on the surface (Fig. 19).
	Chronic	In CSF, ulceration (button ulcers) can be seen in the large intestine (Fig. 20).

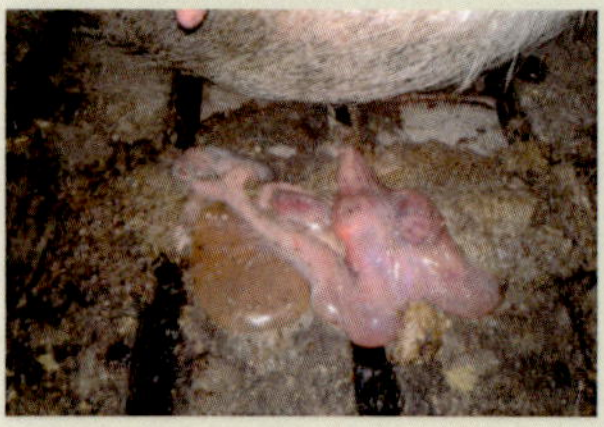

Figure 17. Abortion in an ASF case.

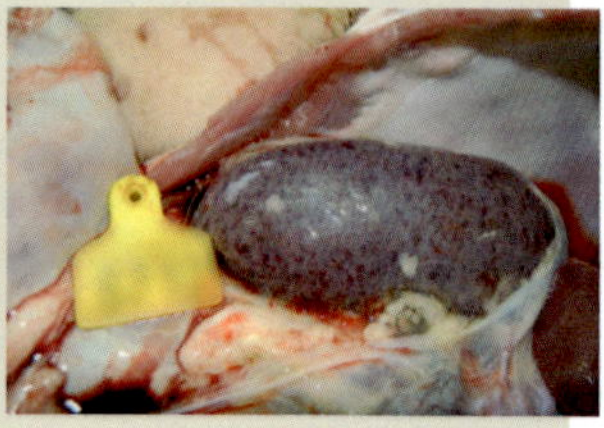

Figure 18. Petechial haemorrhages in the kidney in an ASF case.

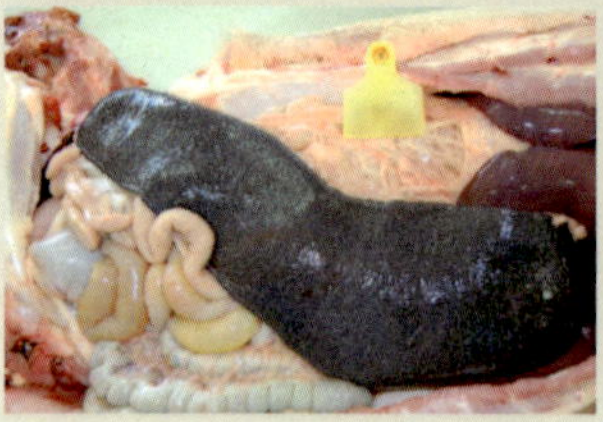

Figure 19. Enlarged spleen in an ASF case.

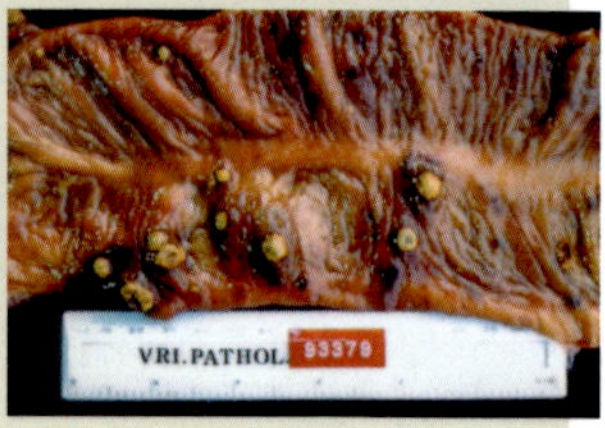

Figure 20. Button ulcers in the large intestine in a CSF case.

MULBERRY HEART DISEASE

Causal agent	Vitamin E/selenium deficiency.
Age group	Postweaning (15–30 kg).
Clinical signs	• Sudden death. Generally, the best pig(s) in the group. • No other clinical signs.
Postmortem lesions	• Large amounts of fluid around the heart and lung. • Haemorrhage and pale areas in the heart muscle. • Fluid in the abdomen with strands of fibrin. • Pale muscle areas in the leg and back. • The liver may be enlarged and mottled with areas of haemorrhage and possible rupture (Fig. 21).

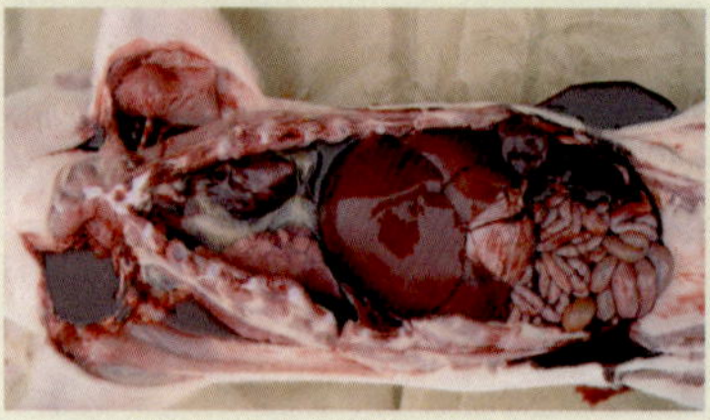

Figure 21. Enlarged and mottled liver with areas of haemorrhage.

PLEUROPNEUMONIA

Causal agent		*Actinobacillus pleuropneumoniae* (APP). There are currently 15 varieties (serovars) described. The severities of the clinical signs differ between the different serovars.
Age group		All ages are susceptible, mainly 20 to 100 kg pigs are affected.
Clinical signs	Peracute	• Sudden illness. May occur in individuals only. • The animals lie down a lot. • High rectal temperature (41.5 °C). • Anorexia (no appetite) and the animals generally do not drink. • The extremities become cyanotic (purple) and are cold to the touch. The cyanosis can spread to the entire body. • Severe breathing difficulties, often with open mouth breathing. Blood-stained froth can be seen at the mouth and nostrils. Death generally occurs within 24 to 48 hours.
	Acute	• Several animals in the group (up to 70%) are depressed and lie down a lot. • High rectal temperatures (40.5 to 41 °C). • Anorexia (no appetite) and the pigs often do not drink either. • Severe respiratory distress, often with a cough and open mouth breathing. • Cyanosis is apparent, particularly if the animal is asked to move. • Vomiting may be seen. • Abortion can occur in sows.
	Subacute	• Intermittent cough in a group of pigs. • Loss of appetite resulting in reduced growth. • Arthritis, endocarditis (heart valve lesions) and abscesses may be seen with APP serovar type 3.
	Chronic	• Intermittent coughing may be heard. • Daily weight gain may not be affected.
	None	Some 25% of pigs at any time may be infected with *A. pleuropneumoniae* without any clinical signs.

Postmortem lesions	Peracute and acute	• Well-demarcated, focal, dark and solid pneumonic areas, particularly in the caudal area of the lung (Fig. 22). Lesions can be found also in the cranial lobe. Lesions may have a red (haemorrhagic) outer edge and a yellow (necrotic, dead) centre (Fig. 23). • Pleurisy, generally very obvious, may be seen adherent to the lesion (Fig. 24). • Fluid around the heart (pericardial effusion) may also be seen.
	Subacute	Pleurisy with no other lung lesions.
	Chronic	There may be a few individuals with pleurisy, but most pigs demonstrate no gross changes.
Other remarks		There are four known toxins: Apx I - strong haemolysin and cytotoxic; Apx II - weak haemolysin and mildly cytotoxic; Apx III - strong cytotoxic. Apx IV is found in all APP strains but has no clinical effect.

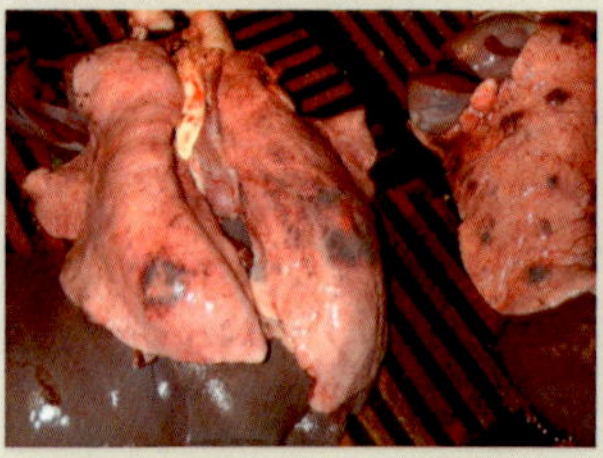

Figure 22. Pleuropneumonia: gross appearance of the lung.

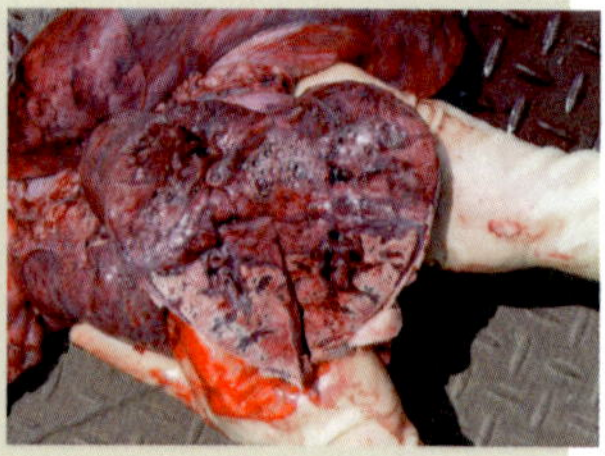

Figure 23. APP: cross-section of the lung showing the yellow necrotic areas.

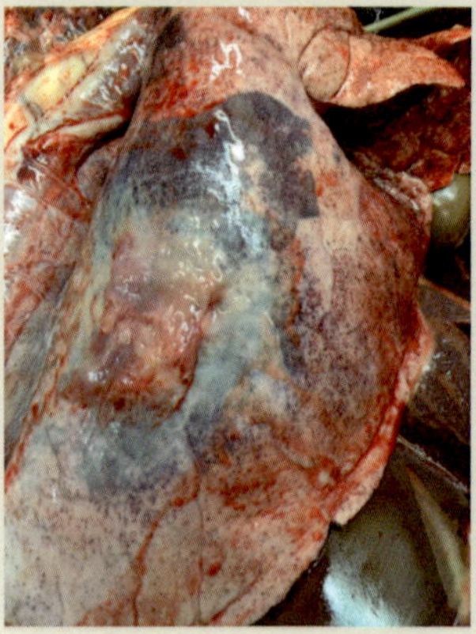

Figure 24. Pleurisy in a pig with APP.

CYSTITIS AND PYELONEPHRITIS

Causal agent	Bacterial infection of the bladder associated with *Actinobaculum suis*, *Escherichia coli* and streptococci, with resulting ascending infection to the kidneys. Environmental factors, such as poor urination and water availability, can also play a role.
Age group	Adult sows, particularly parity 3+.
Clinical signs	• Acute (postservice): urinating blood, off food, collapse, sudden death, hypothermia (Fig. 25). • Chronic (any time): urinating 'smoky' to red/blood urine. Rapid breathing, off food, weakness in hind legs, collapse and death.Unlikely to be a herd problem if the annual death rate in sows less than 5 %.
Postmortem lesions	• Acute catarrhal haemorrhagic ulcerative cystitis (Fig. 26) with thickened bladder wall. Acute changes to the ureterovesical junction. Acute haemorrhagic ureteritis occasionally with occlusion and torsion. • Acute renal failure with haemorrhagic pyelitis. • Chronic and acute catarrhal haemorrhagic cystitis with thickening of the bladder wall. Swollen chronic changes to the ureterovesical junction (Fig. 27). Ureteritis occasionally unilateral. Chronic active interstitial nephritis and pyelonephritis.

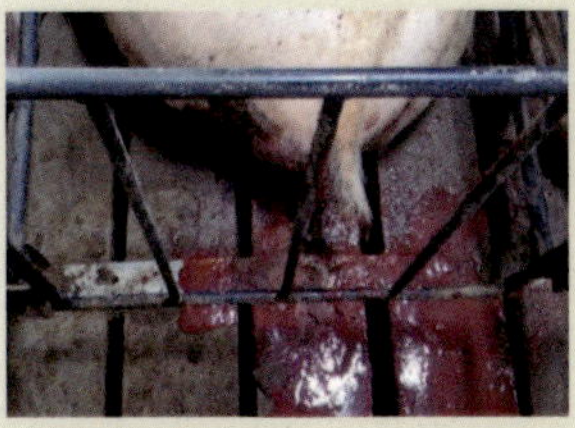

Figure 25. Clinical case of acute pyelonephritis and cystitis.

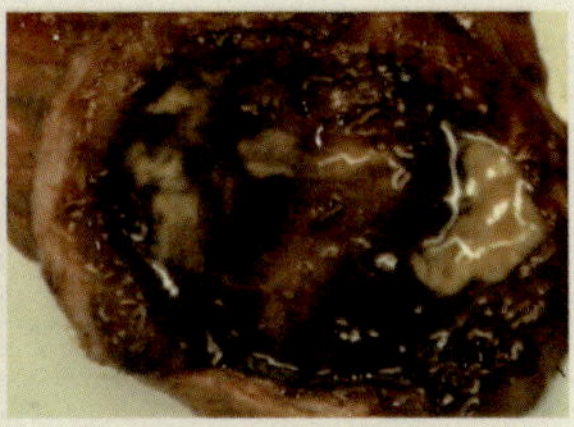

Figure 26. Acute catarrhal haemorrhagic cystitis.

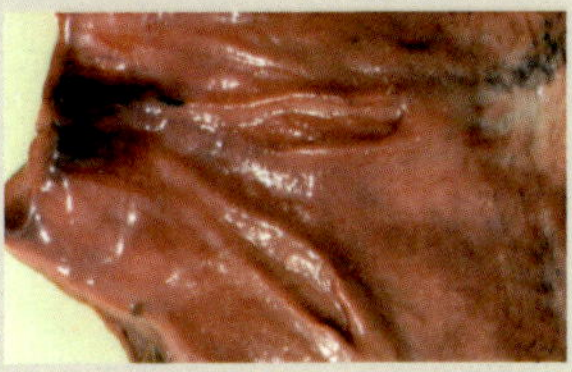

Figure 27. Acute tearing of the ureterovesical junction.

DEFORMITY OF THE HEAD

INFECTIOUS PROGRESSIVE ATROPHIC RHINITIS

Causal agent	Toxigenic forms of *Bordetella bronchiseptica* combined with toxigenic *Pasteurella multocida*, mainly types D and A. Many factors may result in atrophic rhinitis: dust, ammonia, disease agents and genetics. Infectious progressive atrophic rhinitis is the major category of atrophic rhinitis that needs to be controlled on pig farms.
Age group	Any pig weighing more than 10 kg. However, clinical signs usually seen in pigs up to 5 months of age.
Clinical signs	• Virtually all herds are infected with *Bordetella bronchiseptica*; occasional moderate turbinate atrophy is normal. • Sneezing and snuffling in the farrowing area and then throughout the growing phase. • Nose bleeding (epistaxis), usually unilateral. • Snout deformation (Fig. 28). • Growth retardation, which may be up to 7% loss of daily gain. • Turbinate atrophy, possibly with septum deviation. • Tear staining, with brown streaks on the face originating from the medial canthus of the eye. In modern breeds this is quite common without atrophic rhinitis. • Non-immune piglets infected in the first week of life show most severe signs. • Pigs infected after four weeks of age show less severe lesions. • Pigs infected after nine weeks of age show virtually no lesions.
Postmortem lesions	• Distortion of the face. • Atrophy of the nasal turbinates. The atrophy can be scored (Fig. 29), particularly by sawing the nasal cavities at the level between the 1st and 2nd premolar. A straight cut is required, using the lateral commissure of the mouth as reference (Fig. 30).

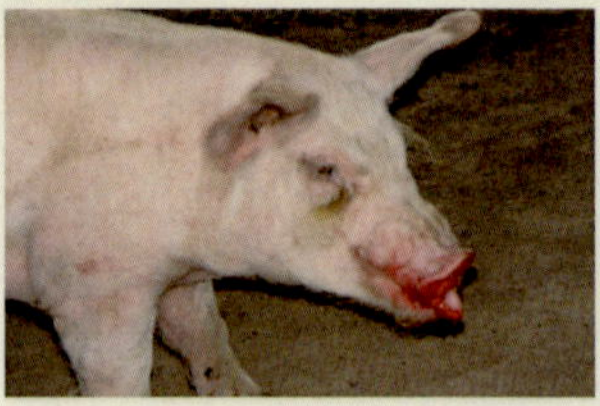

Figure 28. Twisted snouts in a pig.

Figure 29. Atrophic turbinates scores.

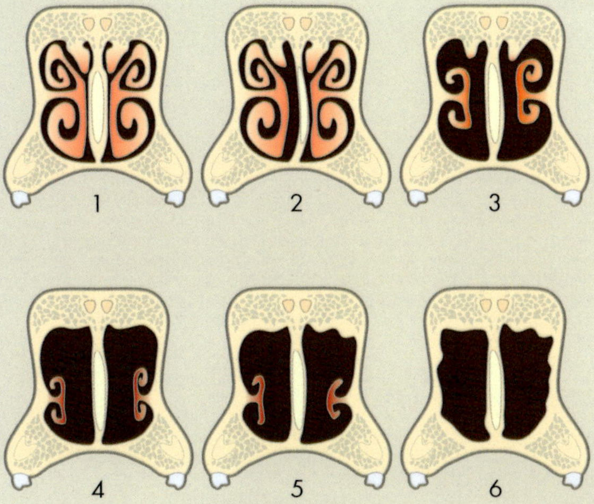

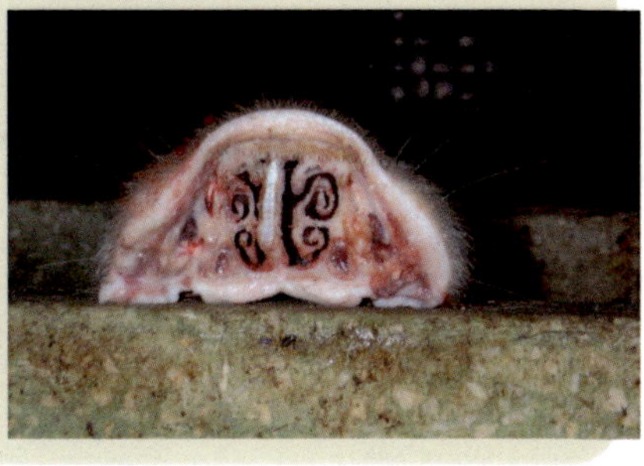

Figure 30. Atrophic turbinates (score 2) and deviated septum.

DIARRHOEA

In piglets, the major causes are: *Clostridium difficile*, clostridial enteritis, coccidiosis, *E. coli* diarrhoea (in the farrowing area and in the nursery), porcine epidemic diarrhoea, rotavirus and transmissible gastroenteritis.

If growing/finishing pigs have diarrhoea, the major cause is, *Brachyspira* colitis, porcine proliferative enteritis (ileitis), salmonellosis and swine dysentery.

CLOSTRIDIUM DIFFICILE ENTERITIS

Causal agent	*Clostridium difficile*, an important gram-positive bacteria pathogen.
Age group	Preweaning, predominately before 10 days of age.
Clinical signs	• Yellow pasty diarrhoea, unresponsive to many antibiotics. • Mild abdominal distension, scrotal oedema in entire males.
Postmortem lesions	• Oedema of the mesocolon, the peritoneal fold covering the colonic loops. • Liquid intestinal contents (Fig. 31). • Histology shows acute multifocal, diffuse erosive colitis with large gram-positive rods on the mucosa.
Other remarks	*Clostridium difficile* is a zoonotic pathogen.

CLOSTRIDIUM PERFRINGENS TYPE C ENTERITIS

Causal agent		*Clostridium perfringens* type C, occasionally A or other types. Often seen in outdoor farming.
Age group		Up to 2–3 week-old piglets.
Clinical signs	Neonatal piglets	• Sudden death. • Haemorrhagic diarrhoea. The anus often bright red. • Other piglets are very weak and pale.
	Older piglets	• Chronic, sometimes intermittent diarrhoea. • Thickened gut walls make food absorption difficult: piglets are emaciated but can be active and alert. • Eventually piglets die.
Postmortem lesions	Neonatal piglets	Intestines full of blood.
	Older piglets	Chronic enteritis with thickened gut walls (Fig. 32).

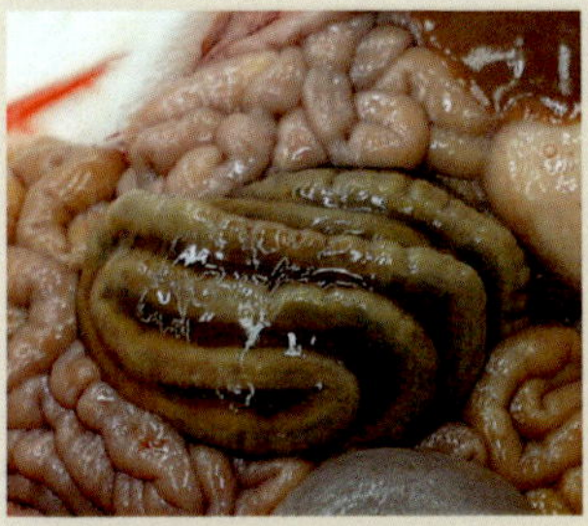

Figure 31. Liquid intestinal contents and moderate oedema of the mesocolon covering the colonic loops.

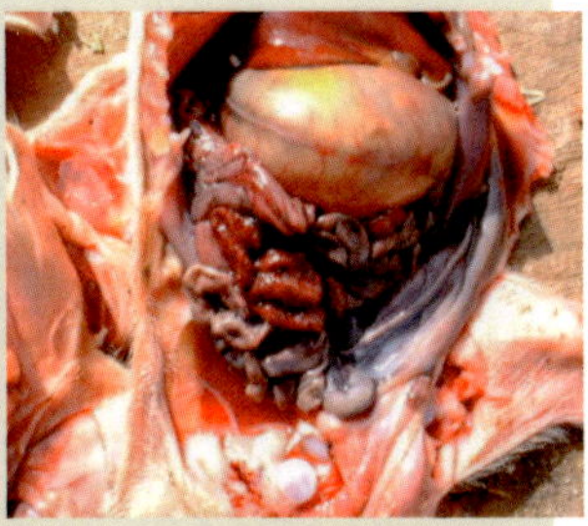

Figure 32. Chronic enteritis with thickened bowels. The intestines have gas bubbles visible on their surface.

COCCIDIOSIS OF PIGLETS

Causal agent	*Cystoisospora suis* is a protozoan parasite that multiplies inside the host cells, mainly in the intestinal tract. It is one of the most common enteric pathogens in neonatal piglets.
Age group	Young piglets (8–15 days of age). Chronic cases can be seen postweaning.
Clinical signs	• Diarrhoea tends to occur in individual pigs from approximately 6 days of age, but most of the litters have diarrhoea at 8–10 days. At the start of the diarrhoea, vomiting may be seen. • Diarrhoea ranges from white to pasty-creamy faeces through to a yellowy watery scour. • Piglets tend to be in poor condition, hairy and growing more slowly than their littermates. • Mortality rates reach 20 % in acute cases. • The diarrhoea is not responsive to antibiotic therapy, excluding sulpha medicines. • Surviving piglets often become unthrifty finishers, as they have little passive immunity and an immature gut. • Failure to recognise the disease leads to increased farrowing house mortality, poorer weaning weights and increased postweaning problems. • Most farms will have coccidiosis at a low (subclinical) level affecting piglet performance.

ENTERIC COLIBACILLOSIS (*E. COLI* PRE AND POSTWEANING DIARRHOEA)

Causal agent		Enterotoxigenic strains of *Escherichia coli*, a gram-negative rod-shaped bacterium. Of the thousands of strains of *E. coli*, the vast majority of *E. coli* are non pathogenic to pigs and may even be beneficial.
Age group		From birth to around 10 days of age. First few weeks postweaning.
Clinical signs	0–3 days	Sudden death, with very few clinical signs. Possibly some diarrhoea.
	3–10 days	Acute watery to chronic diarrhoea, pasty yellow colour. Rapid dehydration and ultimately death (Fig. 33).
	Postweaning	Acute and chronic diarrhoea. Weaners may demonstrate ill-thrift. The diarrhoea progressively leads to dehydration and death.
Postmortem lesions		There may be very few gross pathological findings. • Dilated small intestines filled with yellowish fluid and gas. • Sometimes congestion (dark red colouring) of the stomach or small intestines (Fig. 34). • The intestinal contents will be alkaline.
Other remarks		Various serotypes of *Escherichia coli* are zoonotic.

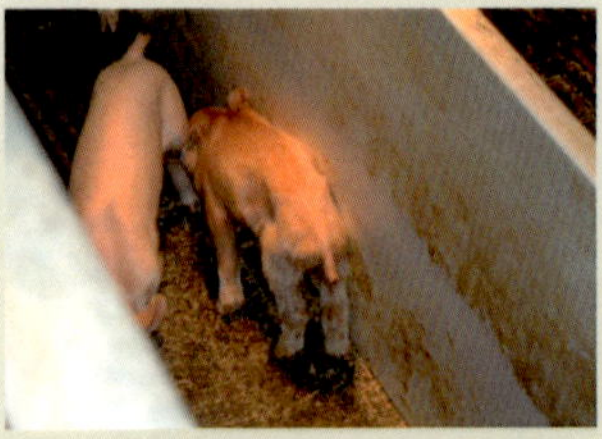

Figure 33. Emaciated piglet with diarrhoea due to *E. coli*.

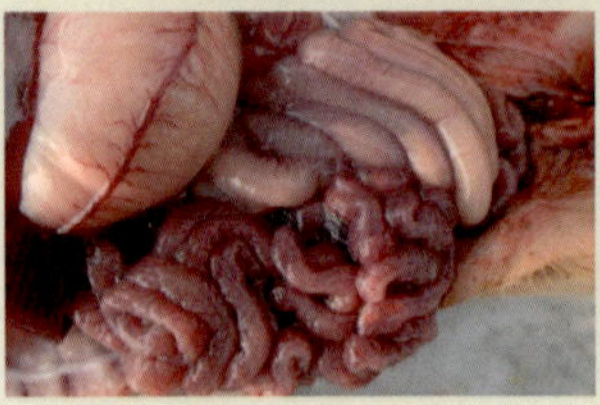

Figure 34. Gross postmortem findings in a pig with enteric colibacillosis: dilated, dark-coloured small intestines and stomach.

PORCINE EPIDEMIC DIARRHOEA (PED)

Causal agent		Porcine epidemic diarrhoea (PED) virus, a coronavirus, type 1 and 2. The virus particles are called "corona" because of their appearance of a crown (as seen by electron microscopy). The disease is reported in Asia, Europe and USA but not in South America or Australia. It clinically resembles transmissible gastroenteritis (TGE), caused by another coronavirus.
Age group		• Type 1 affects all age groups, except suckling piglets. • Type 2 affects all age groups (clinical signs particularly severe in naive piglets).
Clinical signs	Naive herd	• Explosive outbreak. • Mortality of piglets may reach 80 %. • Acute watery diarrhoea in piglets (Fig. 35). • Diarrhoea and vomiting may be seen in all age groups. • Problems persist for 4–6 weeks. • The condition can occur at any time but is more severe in the winter.
	Endemic herd	Little or no problem, as the virus progressively dies out. PED may be more persistent than TGE.
Postmortem lesions		Lesions are mainly found in the small intestines (jejunum and ileum) (Fig. 36). *Villi* atrophy is seen on histology. The pH of the intestinal content is acidic.
Other remarks		• There are a variety of testing methods to help to confirm the diagnosis of different diseases. PED is an example. • Use of sequencing can be vital when investigating the epidemiology of the virus.

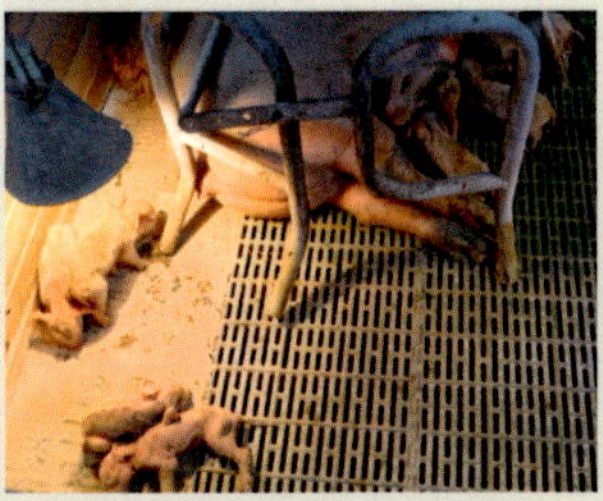

Figure 35. Piglets with porcine epidemic diarrhoea.

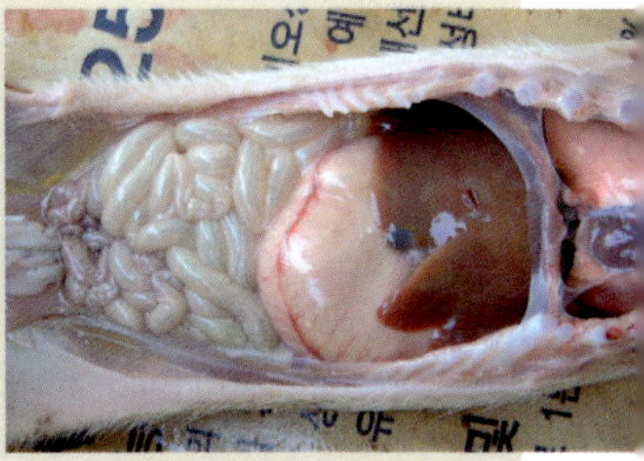

Figure 36. Dilated small intestinal loops in a pig with PED.

ROTAVIRUS DIARRHOEA

Causal agent	Rotavirus, a double-stranded non-enveloped RNA virus. There are many strains. Five types (A-E) are known in pigs, but type A is most common.
Age group	Mainly in young piglets (7 to 14 days of age), rare in pigs over 28 days of age.
Clinical signs	**Lack of colostral immunity** • Severe clinical signs in young pigs (<14 days of age). • Severe profuse diarrhoea that is watery, yellow-whitish with strands of tissue and may also contain undigested food particles ("vomit") (Fig. 37). • Diarrhoea lasts for 3–5 days and mortality may reach 100 %.
	Colostral immunity No clinical signs or mild diarrhoea. The infection may contribute to diarrhoea due to other causes such as *E. coli*.
Postmortem lesions	• Dilated small intestines with watery contents. • Histology will show shortening of the small intestinal *villi*, up to 1/10 length of normal. • The pH of the intestinal contents is acidic (alkaline in *E. coli* diarrhoea). • Findings are more severe in acute cases as the intestinal lesions may recover within 72 hours.

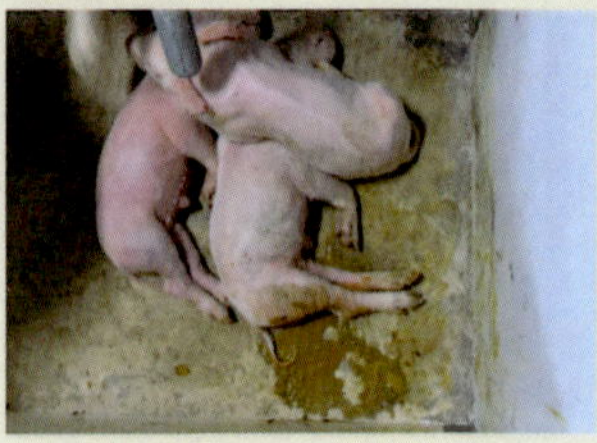

Figure 37. Diarrhoea may also contain undigested food particles.

TRANSMISSIBLE GASTROENTERITIS (TGE)

Causal agent	Transmissible gastroenteritis (TGE) virus, a coronavirus family. Related viruses include: • Porcine respiratory coronavirus (PRCV), a mutant of TGE. • Porcine epidemic diarrhoea (PED) virus. • Haemagglutinating encephalomyelitis virus.
Age group	All ages, although young piglets (<21 days) are the worst affected. The disease spreads rapidly around the farm.

Clinical signs	Initially	• Watery, foul-smelling, yellowish-green diarrhoea. Diarrhoea of unweaned piglets can contain undigested milk particles. • Vomiting and loss of appetite in pigs of all ages. • Young piglets (< 21 days of age) are all affected and generally die. • Weaners become unthrifty. • Growers, finishers and adults are generally mildly affected and will survive if the water supply is adequate. • In smaller herds, outbreaks generally last 3 weeks.
	Chronic	In large herds, the disease can persist for some time, contributing to postweaning diarrhoea.

BRACHYSPIRA COLITIS

Causal agent	*Brachyspira pilosicoli*.
Age group	Mainly affects 10–20 week old growers/finishers (30–90 kg).
Clinical signs (naive herds)	• A non-fatal wasting disease with diarrhoea in growing pigs. • Results in increased days to finish and a reduction in feed efficiency. • Watery/grey brown diarrhoea or loose stools. • The clinical signs are most common 10–14 days after mixing and change of feed (to the grower ration). • 50% of pigs may show transient to persistent watery to mucoid, green-brownish diarrhoea without blood (a "cow pat").
Postmortem lesions	• Inflammation, both acute and chronic of the colon and small intestine. • The spiral colon contains abundant, watery, green or yellow mucoid and frothy contents (Fig. 38). • Erosions in the colonic mucosa may be evident.
Other remarks	*Brachyspira pilosicoli* has a potential zoonotic impact.

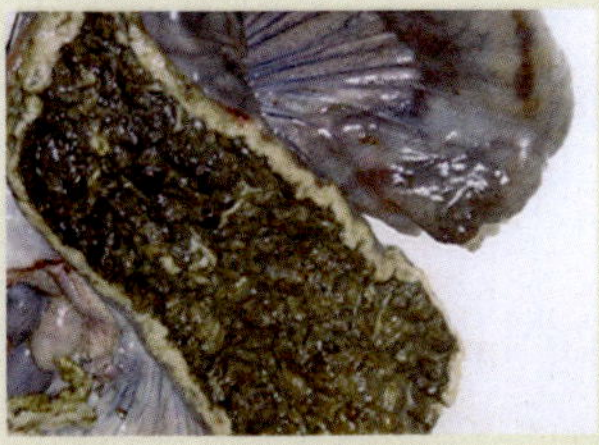

Figure 38. The spiral colon has abundant watery green or yellow mucoid content.

PORCINE PROLIFERATIVE ENTEROPATHY - ILEITIS

Causal agent		*Lawsonia intracellularis*, an intracellular curved bacterium. Several clinical forms of the disease exist, including proliferative haemorrhagic enteropathy (PHE), porcine intestinal adenomatosis (PIA), necrotic or regional ileitis.
Age group		• The acute form occurs in young breeding stock or finishing pigs (>70 kg). • Chronic forms of the disease occur in young growing pigs (20–70 kg). The disease can affect 15 to 50 % of the growing herd.
Clinical signs	Acute form: proliferative haemorrhagic enteropathy (PHE)	• More common in young adults (> 70 kg) • Death (often the first signs seen). • Pale (anaemic) animals. • Depression, reduced appetite and reluctance to move. • Retarded growth. • Watery, dark or bright red diarrhoea (Fig. 39). The hindquarters may be stained with bloody faeces. • Abortion may occur in recovering animals often within 6 days of the onset of clinical signs.
	Chronic forms	More often seen in growing animals (20–70 kg). The clinical signs depend on the extent of the intestinal lesions (Fig. 40).
	PIA Necrotic ileitis Regional Ileitis	• With porcine intestinal adenomatosis (PIA), clinical signs can be very mild with irregular periods of diarrhoea and anorexia. • Animals with necrotic ileitis have more severe clinical signs, with severe loss of condition and often persistent scour. Death is not uncommon. A major effect is the poor food conversion and increased feed costs. In chronically affected herds, the time to slaughter may be extended by up to 14 days. • Animals with regional ileitis also present with severe loss of condition and sometimes a terminal peritonitis.

Postmortem lesions	Postmortem findings are generally restricted to the terminal 50 cm of the small intestine and possibly the first part of the spiral colon and caecum. • PHE: The small intestine and large intestines are dilated, bulging out of the abdomen upon opening, and are filled with blood clots. The colon contains black tarry faeces. The intestinal contents are rarely liquid. • PIA: The intestinal wall is thickened, often with varying degrees of oedema (Fig. 41). The mucosa is folded and may contain sharply defined plaques or marked multiple polyps. • Necrotic ileitis: There is necrosis of the underlying PIA lesion resulting in yellow/grey cheesy masses that adhere tightly to the wall. • Regional ileitis: The lower intestine becomes thickened and rigid, often referred to as hosepipe gut. Ulceration can be seen in the mucosa.

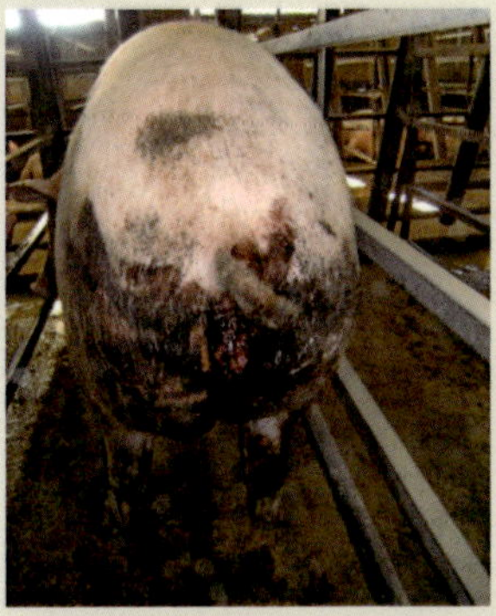

Figure 39. Proliferative haemorrhagic enteropathy: watery, dark or bright red diarrhoea.

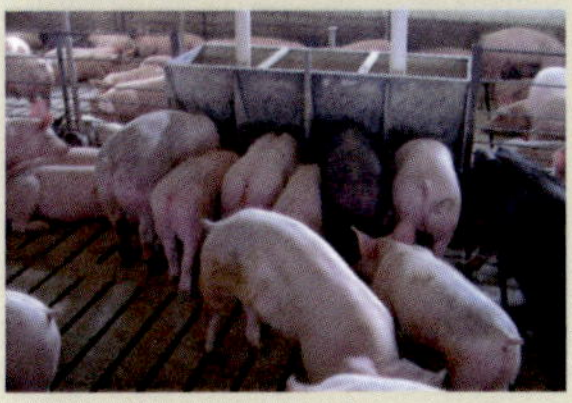

Figure 40. Variable pigs in the growing/finishing pig could be an indication of clinical ileitis.

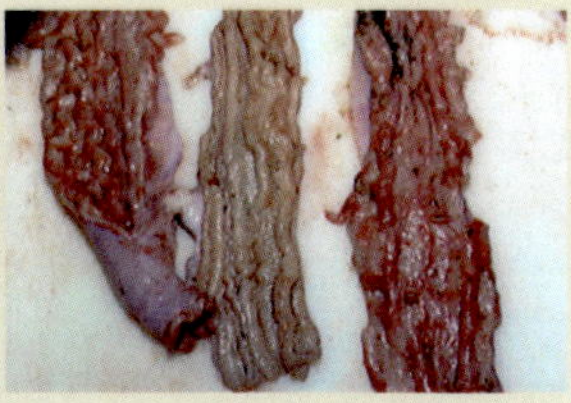

Figure 41. Porcine intestinal adenomatosis: the intestinal wall is thickened often with varying degrees of oedema.

SALMONELLOSIS

Causal agent		*Salmonella* bacteria. There are numerous types of *Salmonella* that can cause a variety of disorders in pigs. The classic salmonella of pigs is *Salmonella enterica* Choleraesuis var Kunzendorf (rare in EU but common in the USA), and *Salmonella enterica* Typhimurium which is much more common worldwide. Clinical signs depend on the type of salmonella infecting the individual pig. Many salmonella serotypes show no clinical signs in the pig.
Age group		All ages can be affected.
Clinical signs	Septicaemia	• Septicaemic salmonellosis is often associated with *S. enterica* Choleraesuis. • This is generally seen in pigs 3 weeks to 5 months of age and is rare in suckling pigs, probably due to intestinal lactobacilli predominance. • Affected piglets are reluctant to move, anorexic, and have a high temperature (40.5–41.6 °C). • Shallow cough. • Huddled together. • A few piglets may be found dead with purple (cyanotic) extremities. • After a couple of days, yellow, often gold-coloured soft faeces/diarrhoea may be seen. • *S. enterica* Choleraesuis can cause pneumonia and diarrhoea in the same pig. • Mortality may be high.
	Enterocolitis	• Enterocolitis is generally associated with *S. enterica* Typhimurium. • Mild wasting and diarrhoea. Initial treatments may be disappointing. • Watery, yellow diarrhoea, initially without blood or mucus (Fig. 42). The diarrhoea may reoccur over the period of a couple weeks. • Mortality is low, and is mainly associated with dehydration and potassium loss. • A few pigs may remain unthrifty and some may develop rectal strictures.

Postmortem lesions	Septicaemia	• Cyanosis of the ears, feet, tail and abdomen (Fig. 43). Enlarged spleen. • The lungs are congested, possibly with interlobular oedema. Jaundice is not uncommon. • There may be miliary white foci of necrosis in the liver. • Necrotic enterocolitis in chronic cases.
	Enterocolitis	• Focal or diffuse necrotic lesions of the colon and caecum, sometimes extending into the small intestine. • Necrotic lesions may also be seen as adherent grey, yellow debris on the red roughened mucosal surface of an oedematous spiral colon and caecum. These may be well demarcated into button ulcers. • The mesenteric lymph nodes are often greatly enlarged. • Intestinal changes may be mild with swollen lymph nodes to a necrotic enteritis that sometimes can be seen through the wall of the intestine (Fig. 44 and Fig. 45). • Lung changes may include blotchy consolidation (Fig. 46).
Other remarks		Many serotypes of *Salmonella* may be zoonotic. Although *Salmonella* can cause infections in live pigs (covered here), the bacteria can also cause contamination of pork and retail products.

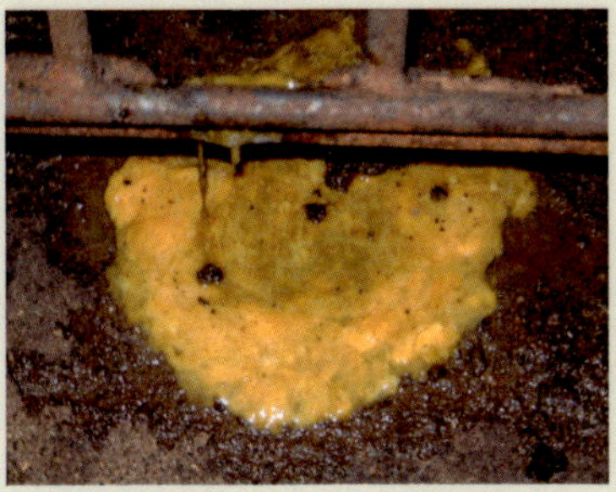

Figure 42. Diarrhoeic faeces of pigs with *Salmonella* enterocolitis are often gold-coloured.

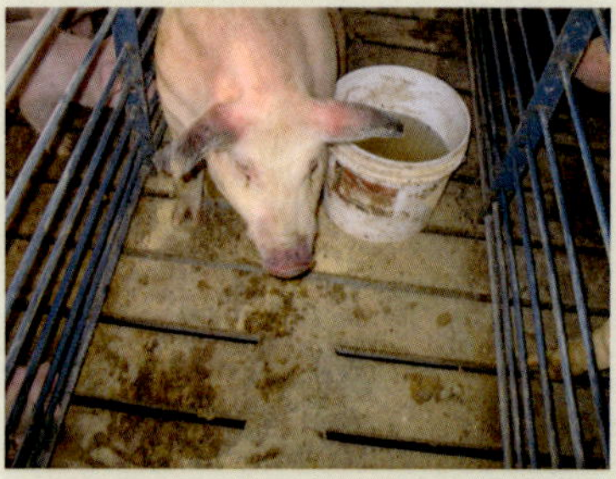

Figure 43. Pigs with *Salmonella* septicaemia may present with cyanosis of the ears, nose and extremities.

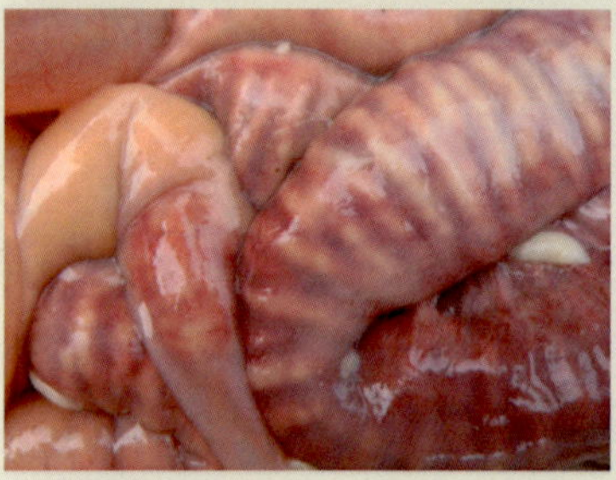

Figure 44. The necrotic lesion in the colon that can be seen through the wall of the intestine.

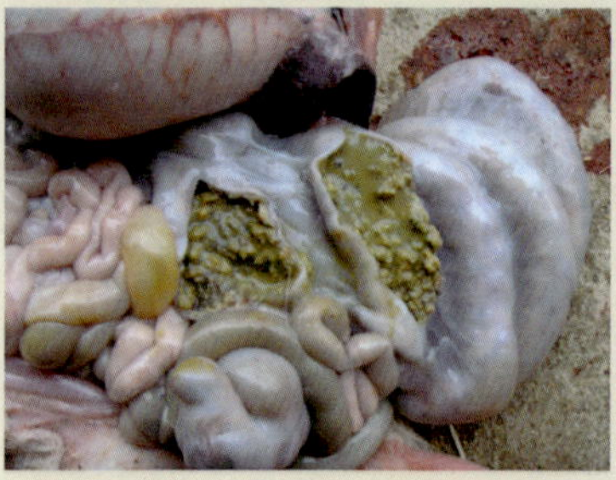

Figure 45. Necrotic enteritis in a pig with *Salmonella* infection.

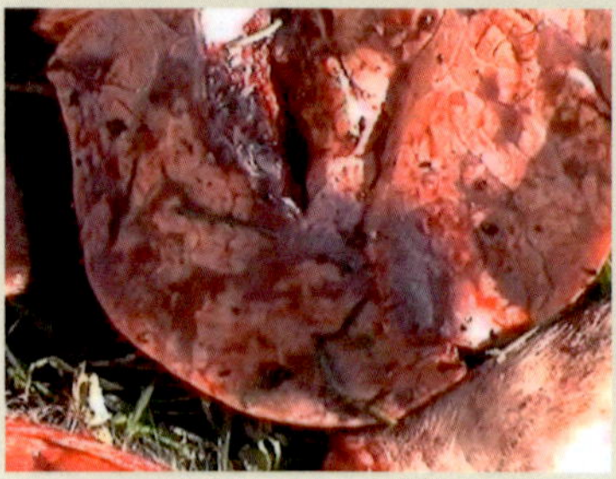

Figure 46. Blotchy consolidation of a lung due to *Salmonella* infection.

SWINE DYSENTERY

Causal agent		*Brachyspira hyodysenteriae*, a bacterium with 12 known serotypes. *Brachyspira hampsonii* may cause similar clinical signs. Even non-pathogenic strains may be associated with dysentery.
Age group		Typically affects pigs from 15 to 70 kg However, in acute outbreaks in naive herds, it can affect all age groups.
Clinical signs	Naive herds	• Death of one or two pigs before other pigs show any signs. • Diarrhoea, with or without blood, of varying severity, sometimes with large amounts of mucus and later with flecks of blood. A thorough search of the pen normally reveals the presence of blood and mucus in some places. • Rapid loss of condition in some pigs; pigs may look "hairy". • Up to 50% of pigs are clinically affected. • FCR becomes poorer with a loss of 0.6 while disease present with extension of finishing by 20 days.
	Established herds	• Dehydration, a painful abdomen. • Some pigs may be weak and uncoordinated. • Cyclic disease, reappearing at 3–4 week intervals.
Postmortem lesions		• Confined to the large bowel: caecum, colon and rectum. • Hyperaemia (reddening) and oedema of the walls of the large intestine. • Submucosal glands of the colon may be more prominent and appear white. • The mucosa is usually covered by mucus and fibrin with flecks of blood and the colonic contents are soft to watery (Fig. 47).

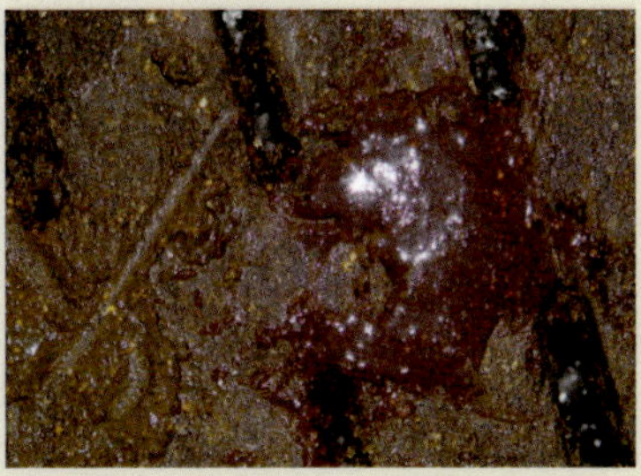

Figure 47. A severe case of dysentery with extensive bleeding into the colon.

VULVAR DISCHARGE IN SOWS

Causal agent	14 to 21 day postservice vulvar discharge following infection of the genital tract late in oestrus. There is no specific causal agent, although *Escherichia coli*, *Staphylococcus*, *Streptococcus* and *Klebsiella* are often isolated from swabs.
Clinical signs	Creamy cheesy discharge from the vulva 14–21 days after mating, without blood (Fig. 48). The sow subsequently returns to oestrus at 18–24 days postmating. It is essential to confirm the sow returns and is not pregnant.

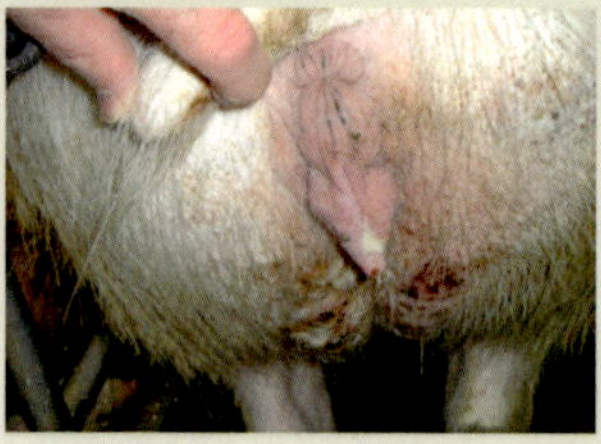

Figure 48. Sow showing 14–21 day postservice vulval discharge.

ITCHY PIGS

MANGE (SCABIES)

Causal agent	*Sarcoptes scabiei* var. *suis*, a parasitic mite that burrows into skin and causes mange (scabies).
Age group	All age groups are affected, although sows and growing pigs most often exhibit the characteristic clinical signs.
Clinical signs	• Scratching: piglets may be uncomfortable and have intermittent body scratching. • A few weeks later the weaned and growing pig demonstrate persistent itching and rubbing. • Excessive earwax, sometimes forming plaques. • Chronic lesions may occur with thickened skin, hair loss and abrasions, especially behind the ear and at the base of the tail (Fig. 49).
Other remarks	• Worldwide distribution (70 % or more herds infected). • The female mite lays about 1 to 3 eggs a day in the skin, mainly in the soft tissues of the inside of the ear. The adult female lives for about a month and produces some 30 to 40 eggs in a lifetime. There may be as many as 18,000 mites per gram of ear skin. • The eggs hatch after 5 days. The mite larvae moult into nymphs, which moult into adults after 10 to 15 days. The mites remain on the pig during the entire life cycle.

LAMENESS

BUSH FOOT/SWOLLEN FOOT/FOOT ROT

Cause	Infection enters the foot through a number of routes: • Following a puncture or trauma wound to the lower leg. • Toes can become trapped and torn in slats (Fig. 50). • Open wounds are not uncommon following abrasion from rough floors.
Clinical signs	The infection can spread from the coronary band into the foot resulting in severe necrosis (Fig. 51) of the internal tissues, including osteomyelitis.
Other remarks	Treatment must be vigorous. Failure to respond quickly usually leads to euthanasia. In the early stages, move the pig to a bedded hospital area and treat vigorously. Review flooring, particularly slat quality. Once the infection has penetrated the internal tissues, treatment is generally pointless.

FOOT-AND-MOUTH DISEASE

Causal agent	There are several diseases that can cause blisters on feet and snout: • Foot-and-mouth disease, caused by a picornavirus (Aphthovirus). • Vesicular stomatitis, caused by a rhabdovirus (Vesiculovirus). • Other viruses, also picornaviruses: Swine vesicular disease; Seneca Valley virus; Vesicular exanthema and San Miguel Seal Lion virus. Foot-and-mouth disease (FMD) is the definitive disease, the other diseases have signs that may be confused with FMD.
Age group	Pigs of all ages can be affected.
Clinical signs	• Incubation period 1 to 5 days (up to 21 days). • Fever to 40.5 °C. • Skin around the snout, lips, tongue, inside the mouth, around the coronary band and the soft skin on the feet becomes whiter. • Vesicles (blisters) develop here as well as on the sow's teats. Mouth lesions are not always obvious in the pig. • Vesicles rupture up to 24 hours after development. If no secondary infection occurs, healing is rapid. • The animals are lame. • The hoof may become detached (Fig. 52), revealing the painful raw tissues underneath. The hoof can regrow, but is often deformed. This can take several weeks. • The disease affects nearly all susceptible animals, but few animals will die specifically with the disease.

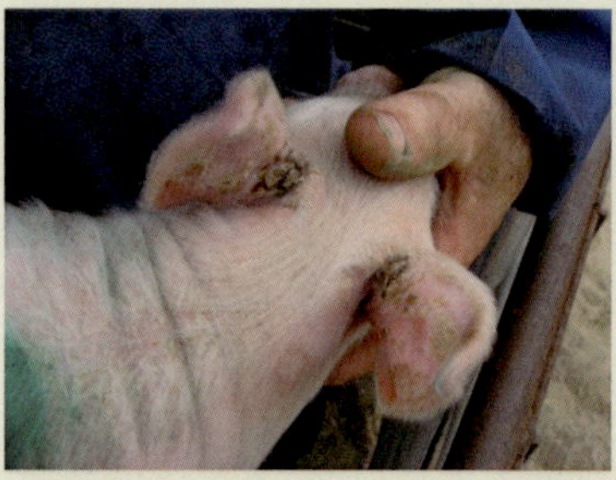

Figure 49. Itchy pig with thickened skin behind the ears.

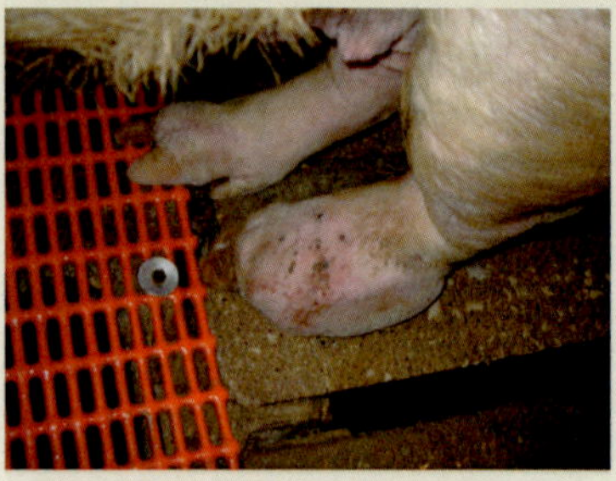

Figure 50. Swollen foot.

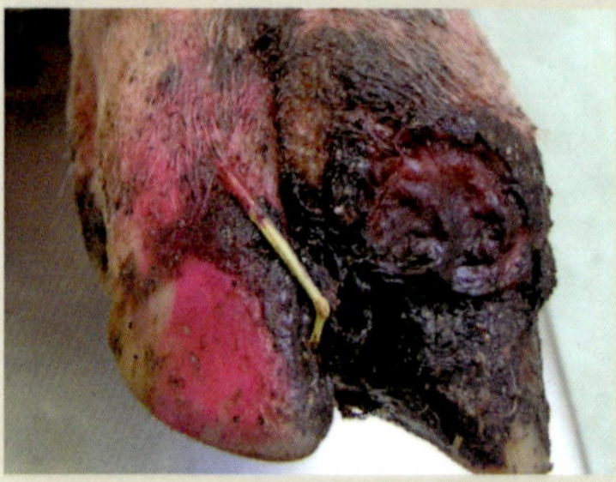

Figure 51. Necrosis of the foot.

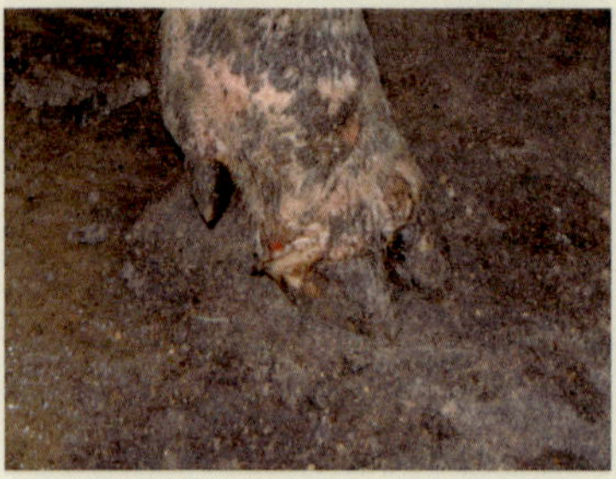

Figure 52. Horn separation of the foot of a pig with FMD.

JOINT ILL

Causal agent	Mainly *Streptococcus suis* type I bacteria although many other species of streptococci can be involved. *Trueperella pyogenes* may also play a role.
Age group	Piglets.
Clinical signs	Acute swelling of one or more of the joints, piglets may be acutely lame (Figs. 53 and 54). With time, the joint swellings resolve.
Postmortem lesions	A purulent tenosynovitis which can be very severe (Fig. 55). Multiple joints may be affected.

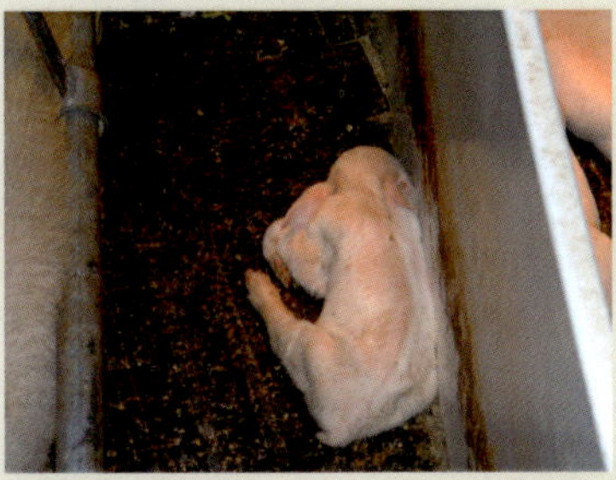

Figure 53. Large infected shoulder joint.

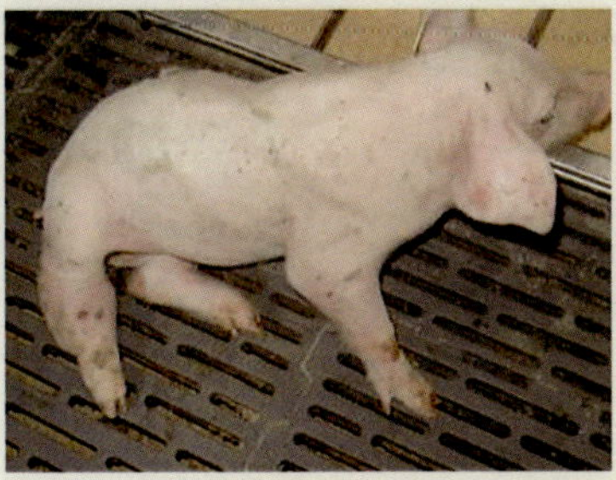

Figure 54. Abscess on the hock joint.

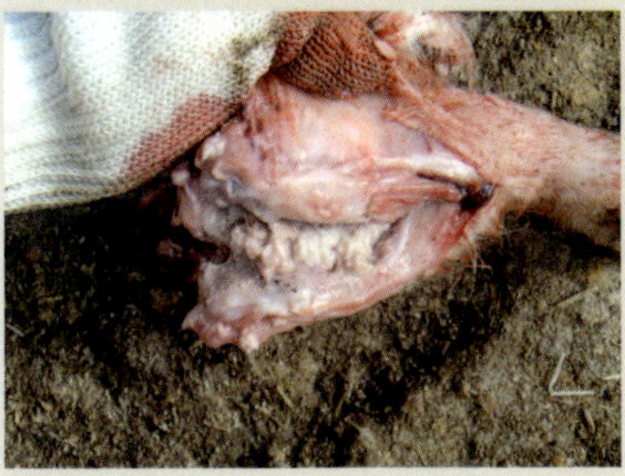

Figure 55. Purulent tenosynovitis.

SPLAY LEG (STRADDLERS, MYOFIBRILLAR HYPOPLASIA)

Causal agent	Environmental factors: • Slippery floors especially behind the sow. • Piglets staying wet and cold too long. • Low birth weight piglets. • Stressed sows at farrowing more prone to deliver splay leg piglets. Mycotoxins: • Zearalenone (F2) toxin may be associated with increased incidence. Genetics: • In some cases there is a genetic component (more common in Landrace than in Large White).
Age group	Newborn piglets within hours of birth. Males are more commonly affected.
Clinical signs	Splayed back legs and occasionally front legs (Fig. 56). This seriously affects the piglet's ability to dry, suckle and get out of the way of the sow, leading to increased preweaning mortality.

MYCOPLASMA ARTHRITIS

Causal agent	*Mycoplasma hyosynoviae bacteria*. The environment plays a role in the clinical expression of *Mycoplasma* arthritis.
Age group	Growers to young adults. Typically, the condition is seen in a new group of gilts/boars 10–14 days after arrival on the farm.
Clinical signs	• Sudden lameness of the legs, often with one hind leg more severely lame than the other. • Swollen joints. • Few outward signs on the leg apart from lameness.
Postmortem lesions	Non-purulent synovitis of the affected joints (Fig. 57).

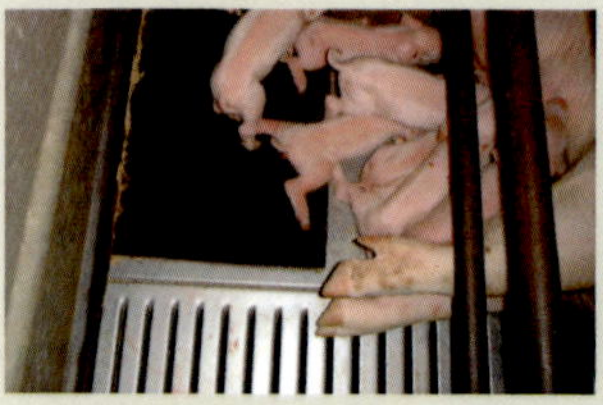

Figure 56. Piglet with splayed back legs.

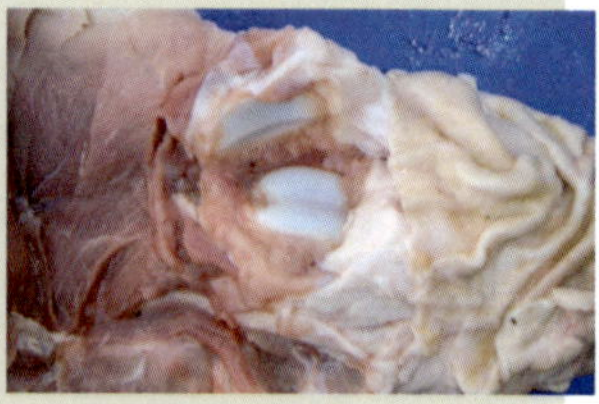

Figure 57. Synovitis of an elbow joint.

FEMORAL HEAD FRACTURE – EPIPHYSIOLYSIS

Causal agent	Trauma in combination with *epiphysiolysis*, a specific form of osteochondrosis affecting the neck of the femur. Often occurs after trauma (bullying, pushing through a narrow doorway, mating).
Age group	Gilts.
Clinical signs	Sudden unilateral hind limb lameness with collapse of the gluteal (hip) muscles, often on one side (Fig. 58). There is no effective treatment.

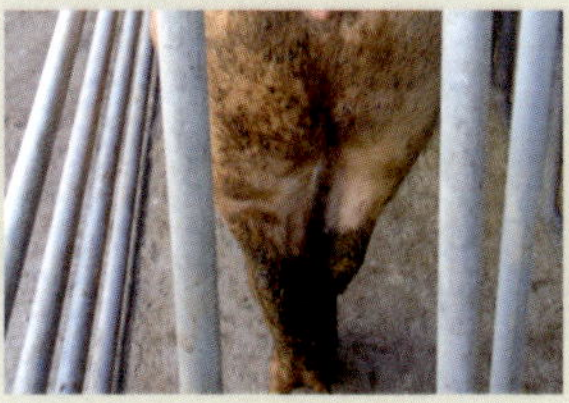

Figure 58. Lame young sow with epiphysiolysis. Note the crosslegged stance.

UDDER PROBLEMS

UDDER OEDEMA

Causal agent	Poor management: common in overweight sows that receive too high a feed plane while pregnant, in particular at the end of pregnancy.
Age group	Sows and gilts. Udder oedema may be seen in the dry/gestating sow 20 days prior to farrowing.
Clinical signs	• Build-up of fluids in the mammary gland with little or no milk let-down. • Painful milk glands, which may interfere with locomotion. • Palpation of the gland will reveal oedema (when a thumb is pressed into the udder, the depression will take a long time to disappear). • Piglets attempting to use the affected teats will not thrive and may require fostering.

ACUTE MASTITIS

Causal agent	Mainly *E. coli* but staphylococci and/or streptococci may also be involved. Accurate diagnosis of the causal agent is complicated by the difficulty in obtaining a suitable sample to investigate.
Clinical signs	• Affected sows are obviously ill and probably toxic (may have discoloured ears). • The udder is hard and reddened particularly in the infected area (Fig. 59). • Fever (40–42 °C). • Only one mammary gland in the chain may be affected.

CHRONIC MASTITIS

Causal agent	Associated with a range of bacteria such as *Staphylococcus*, *Streptococcus*, *Trueperella pyogenes* and *Actinobacillus suis*.
Clinical signs	• Large, often multiple, lumps in the mammary gland (Fig. 60), classically first seen at the end of lactation or in the newly weaned sow. • Usually no other clinical signs. • The infected gland will be non-functional. Once observed, there is no effective treatment.

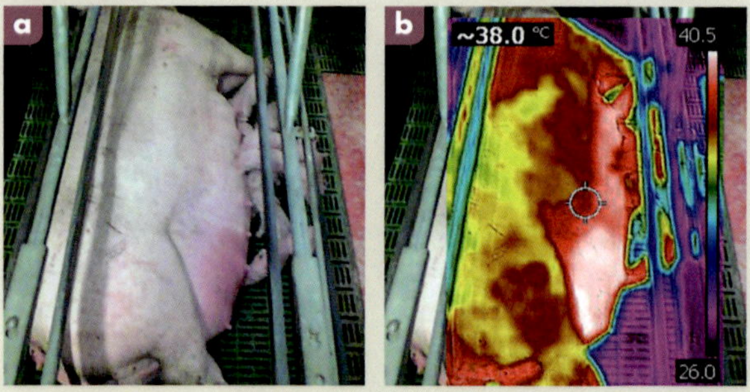

Figure 59. Acute mastitis (a). Note the hot udder which is indicated by white in the right infrared picture (b).

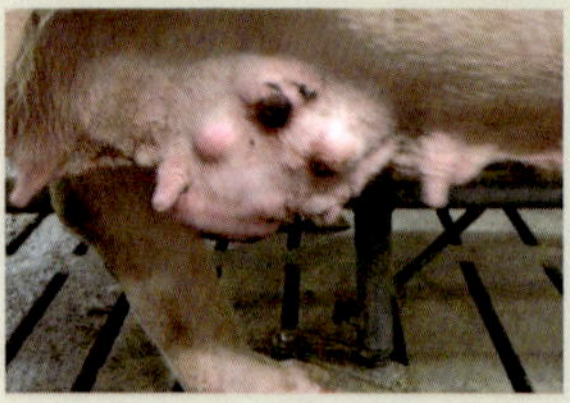

Figure 60. Chronic mastitis.

NEUROLOGICAL PROBLEMS

AUJESZKY'S DISEASE (PSEUDORABIES)

Causal agent		Aujeszky's disease (AD, pseudorabies) virus, a herpes virus. Several countries are free of Aujeszky's disease.
Age group		All age groups, mainly in naive herds. Few clinical signs in herds where the virus has established.
Clinical signs	Neonatal piglets	• A range of severe central nervous signs, ranging from fits to severe incoordination. The piglets may be "sitting like a dog" due to posterior paralysis. • Mortality is high.
	Weaned pigs	• Less central nervous signs, more respiratory signs. • Respiratory diseases often associated with secondary infections. • Animals can waste and suffer ill-thrift and are often stunted.
	Growing pigs	Less central nervous signs, more respiratory signs. The degree of respiratory disease depends on secondary infections.
	Adults	Reproductive signs predominate (abortion; stillborn or weak piglets if the sow is infected close to term).
Postmortem lesions		Gross lesions are often absent or minimal. • A serous to fibrinous rhinitis and necrotic tonsillitis is common. • Respiratory lesions of complicated pneumonia • The liver and spleen typically have yellow-white necrotic foci (2–3 mm). • A necrotic placentitis and endometritis may be observed. • In aborted piglets there may be necrotic lesions in the lungs, liver, spleen and tonsils.
Other remarks		• The pig is the natural host for AD. • In other animals, the disease either causes no problems or is invariably fatal. • In cats, rats and mice the disease kills rapidly and this can be important in diagnosis. Dogs show rabid signs, hence the name pseudorabies. Cattle and sheep (rarely horses) present with a "mad itch". • Aujeszky's disease does not affect man.

MENINGITIS

Causal agent		*Streptococcus suis* II. Other types of *S. suis* may also be associated with meningitis in pigs. The organism lives on the tonsils and upper respiratory tract of normal healthy pigs. Several other bacteria can cause also meningitis, including *Haemophilus parasuis*. Septicaemic *Escherichia coli* (bowel oedema) will cause similar clinical findings but no meningitis.
Age group		All ages, although meningitis classically occurs between 3–60 kg. *H. parasuis* in naive finishing and adult pigs can cause a devastating acute fatal meningitis.
Clinical signs	Acute	• The pig becomes uncoordinated often with uncontrolled eye movements. • Rectal temperature is increased to 40–41 °C. • As the condition progresses, the pig will fall over and thrash with all four legs on the floor (Fig. 61). • The pig may hurt itself during these thrashing movements. • Death occurs quickly especially if the pig is stressed. In the farrowing house, the condition can then be misdiagnosed as having been crushed by the sow. • If treatment is late a neurologically damaged pig may result.
Other remarks		*Streptococcus suis* is a zoonotic pathogen.

WATER DEPRIVATION/SALT POISONING

Causal agent	Management mistake. The disease may be associated with high salt (NaCl) levels in drinking water (> 7000 ppm).
Age group	All ages. Classically seen in the nursery.
Clinical signs	Drinking supply off or at least inadequate. • Several dead pigs. • Pig adopts sitting dog position, staring into space. • Twitching, developing into a seizure every 5 minutes. Pigs may walk aimlessly and frequently fall over or appear blind and press their heads against the wall. • Pigs may be very dirty especially if the building is hot.
	Once the water source is restored, the pigs will crowd around drinkers (Fig. 62). Drinking can be excessive. • Pigs suddenly fall over, show tremor and have fits. Several pigs may die.

CONGENITAL TREMOR, SHAKING PIGLET

Causal agent	Different possible causes, including viruses (including classical swine fever virus, Aujeszky's disease virus), genetics ("Landrace trembles", "Saddleback tremors") and toxins. Congenital tremor A-II is a pestivirus.
Age group	Newborn piglets. The problem classically occurs in naive gilt litters from newly introduced stock.
Clinical signs	• Newborn piglets tremble all over. They may be unable to walk and often are unable to suckle efficiently. Sometimes the trembling is noticeably reduced when the piglet is asleep. • Once attached to the teat by the stockperson, the piglet will suckle vigorously, but once let go the piglet will often shake itself away from the teat. • Increased preweaning mortality (crushed by sow) and diseases. • Increased lameness from trauma, outbreaks of scour. • Due to the lack of suckling, the piglet will have problems ingesting sufficient colostrum. Mortality rates of 75 to 100 % are common. • In surviving piglets, the clinical signs subside with age. An occasional tremble over the ears and muscles on the back (fasciculation) is noticeable if the animal relaxes.

BOWEL OEDEMA, OEDEMA DISEASE

Causal agent	Certain serotypes of *Escherichia coli* bacteria that produce a powerful toxin (STx2e toxin).
Age group	2 weeks postweaning (nursery pigs).
Clinical signs	• Sudden death 2 weeks postweaning (sometimes the only sign). • Diarrhoea. • Neurological signs: leg paralysis, splay-leg, circling and severe ataxia (staggering). • Swollen eyelids (Fig. 63).
Postmortem lesions	• Oedema of the mesocolon (Fig. 64), stomach, eyelids and forehead. • Note no meningitis.

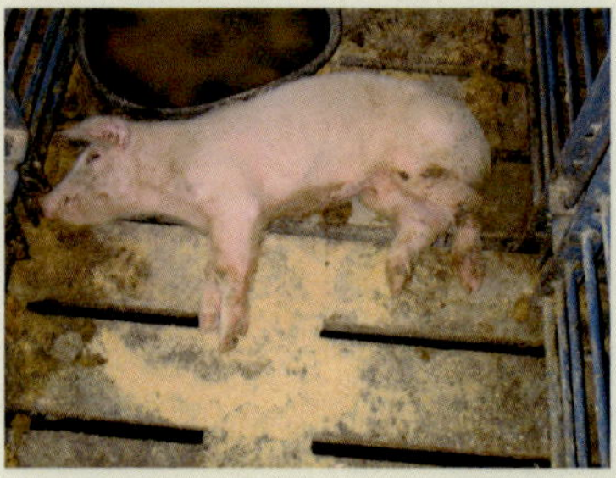

Figure 61. Meningitis in a weaner. Note the paddling indicated by the cleared patch in the feed on the floor.

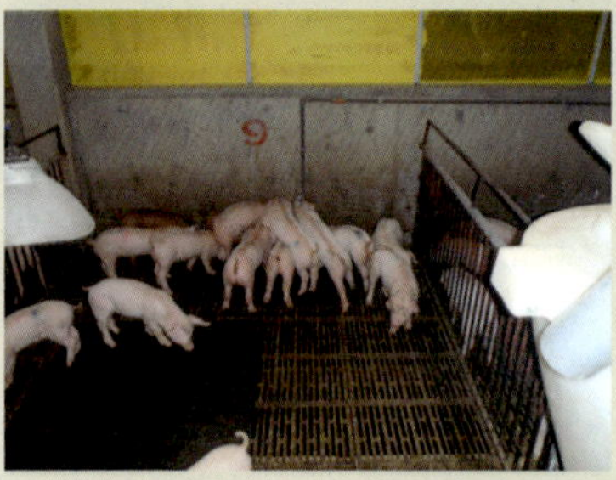

Figure 62. Pigs crowding around drinker.

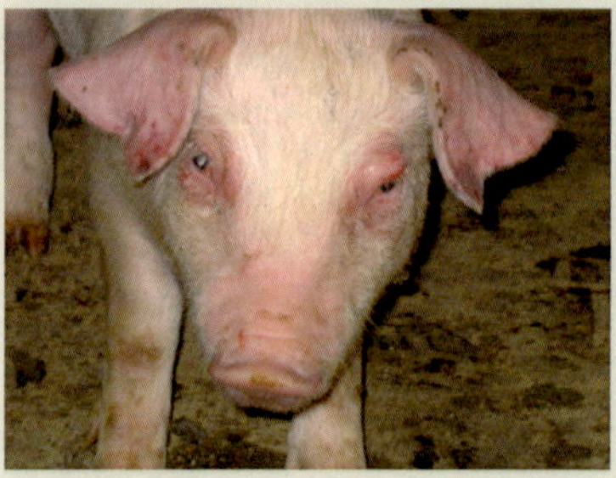

Figure 63. Dying weaner with swollen eyelids due to oedema disease.

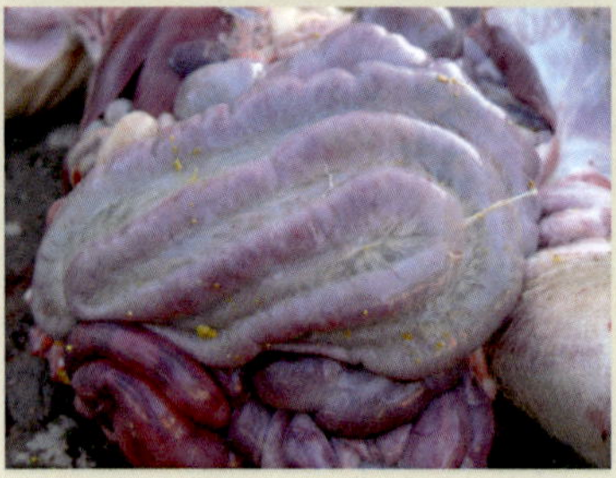

Figure 64. Oedema in the loops of the spiral colon.

"POOR", UNTHRIFTY PIGS

GLÄSSER'S DISEASE

Causal agent		*Haemophilus parasuis* alone or a combination with various streptococci and *Mycoplasma hyorhinis*. *H. parasuis* and many of the other 'pathogens' are normal inhabitans of the nasopharynx.
Age group		All ages, however weaned pigs seem most susceptible.
Clinical signs	Naive herds (very rare)	• Acute meningitis. This is normally seen when a naive adult is introduced to a normal herd. • Within 48 hours, the adult demonstrates severe pneumonia, depression, anorexia, high rectal temperature 42 °C). • Terminally, the animal shows incoordination, prostration, meningitis and dies. • Death can occur very quickly after arrival.
	Normal herds (acute)	Clinical signs are usually sudden and often affect the "better" pig: • Depression, anorexia, the rectal temperature rises to 40.5 °C. • Cyanosis may appear on the extremities. The animal may appear as if walking is painful. • Terminally, meningitis may be seen. • Sometimes, no signs are seen (sudden death).
	Chronic	• Poor blood supply to the ears (pigs may lose part of the ear). • Piglets who fade and die (wasting) or grow very poorly. • Death in late growers.
Postmortem lesions		Polyserositis, or inflammation of the serosal membranes. The postmortem signs depend on the organ affected. The following organs are covered by a serosal membrane: • Heart: pericarditis with fibrin strands ("tags") and fluid around the heart (Figs. 65 and 66). • Lungs: extensive pleurisy (Fig. 66). • Intestines and abdomen: peritonitis (Fig. 66) • Joints: synovitis and arthritis (swollen joints). • Brain: meningitis.

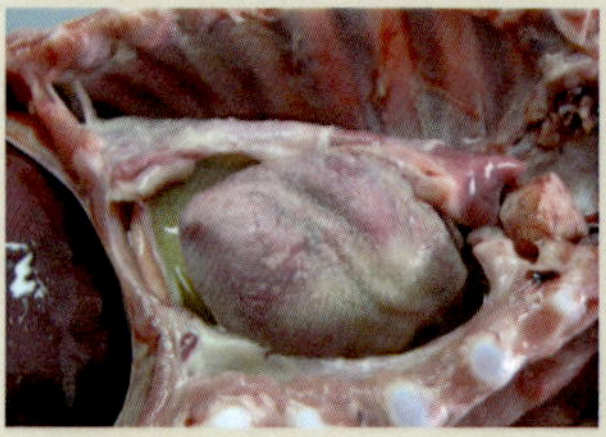

Figure 65. Chronic pericarditis.

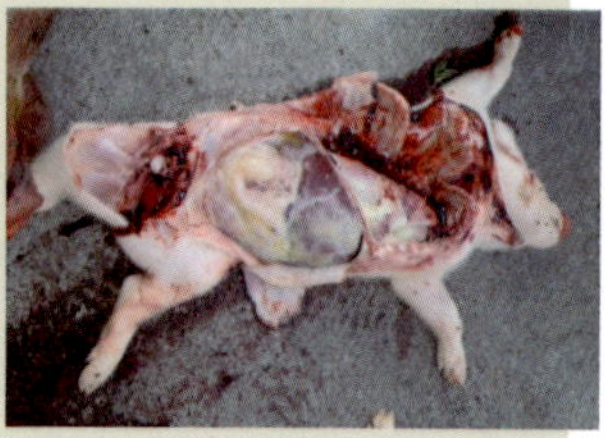

Figure 66. Glässer's polyserositis (pericarditis, pleurisy and peritonitis).

PASTEURELLOSIS AND STREPTOCOCCI INFECTIONS

Causal agent		*Pasteurella multocida* and various species of streptococci, typically *S. suis*, both bacteria.
Age group		Growing and finishing pigs.
Clinical signs	Acute form	Most commonly associated with *P. multocida* serotype B. • Dyspnoea, laboured breathing, "thumping" (abdominal breathing), high fever (up to 42.2 °C), prostration and finally death. • Purple discoloration of the abdomen.
	Subacute	Pleuritis, coughing and difficulty in breathing.
	Chronic	• Generally affects pigs from 10–16 weeks of age (25–50 kg). • Occasional cough, thumping and little or no fever. In chronic cases the pig can lose a lot of weight. • Poor or no growth, with serious consequences for the pig flow.
Postmortem lesions		*Pasteurella* is found in the enzootic pneumonia complex with lesions resulting in consolidation of the cranial lung lobes: • Pleurisy and abscesses in severe cases (Fig. 67). • In association with viral agents (e.g. PRRSv or swine influenza), *Pasteurella* can produce lesions closely resembling enzootic pneumonia, even in EP-negative herds. Water deprivation and high ammonia concentrations can produce very similar gross pathology when combined with *Pasteurella* infection.

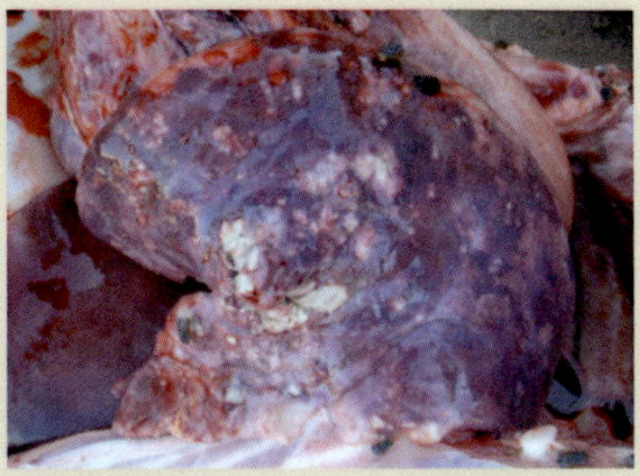

Figure 67. Streptococci are commonly associated with pulmonary abscesses.

POSTWEANING ILL-THRIFT, PERIWEANING FAILURE-TO-THRIVE SYNDROME (PFTS)

Causal agent	Starvation. The piglets fail to learn to eat and drink when weaned.
Age group	Immediately postweaning. Not dependent on weaning age but more common when piglets are weaned before 17 days of age.
Clinical signs	• Severe emaciated weaners 10–15 days postweaning (Fig. 68). • Weaners are gaunt, dehydrated, lethargic and often uncoordinated. • Affected weaners often exhibit signs of vice (penile sucking, sham nursing).
Postmortem lesions	• The stomach and small intestines will be empty of food. • Sometimes, the stomach is filled with fluid and possibly just straw (if housed on bedding). However, the weaner may have just figured out how to eat. • Emaciated carcases, absence of body fat • The superficial inguinal lymph nodes may be more prominent. • Pale liver. • Histological changes in the small intestine include villus atrophy and fusion.

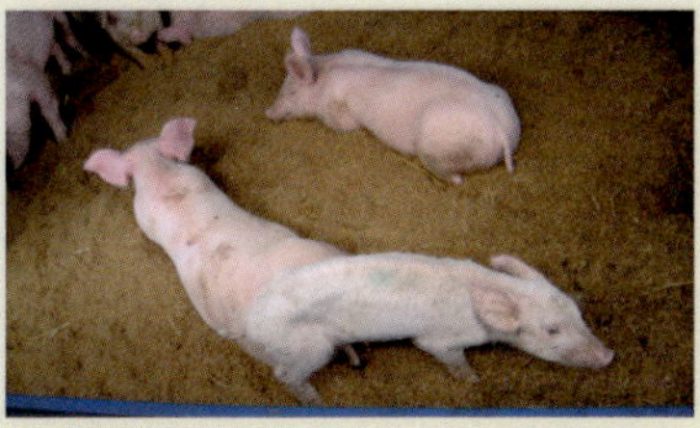

Figure 68. Emaciated weaner with PFTS.

PORCINE CIRCOVIRUS SYSTEMIC DISEASE (PCV-SD)

Causal agent		Porcine Circovirus systemic disease (PCV-SD) is a multifactorial disease associated with porcine circovirus type 2 found in high numbers.
Age group		All age groups • Weaners: PCV-SD and PMWS. • Growers: PCV-SD, PMWS, PDNS and granulomatous enteritis. • Adults: abortion (foetal death) and without other clinical signs.
Clinical signs	Weaner	The problem will generally present as a single batch or a series of batches but only while the management/diseases problems persist. • PCV-SD: 15–60 kg pigs present with acute wasting, generally within 4 days becoming extremely emaciated. Surrounding pigs are normal and then waste rapidly. • Mortality generally extremely high (20 % or more). Death is associated with other infections already on the farm.
	Grower	• Growers present with porcine dermatitis and nephropathy syndrome (PDNS) (Fig. 69), even though the role of PCV2 or PCV3 in PDNS is not determined. • Granulomatous enteritis may be associated with PCV2 and result in ileitis and wasting disorders.
	Adult sows	• Abortion, mummification and stillborn piglets. • Reproductive effects are minimal/non-existent. Could play a role in stillbirth, mummification, embryonic death and infertility (SMEDI) syndromes.
Other remarks		Most pigs and almost all pig farms are infected with PCV2 without any clinical signs. If the pigs are severely stressed with primary pathogens or due to management problems clinical signs can be severe.

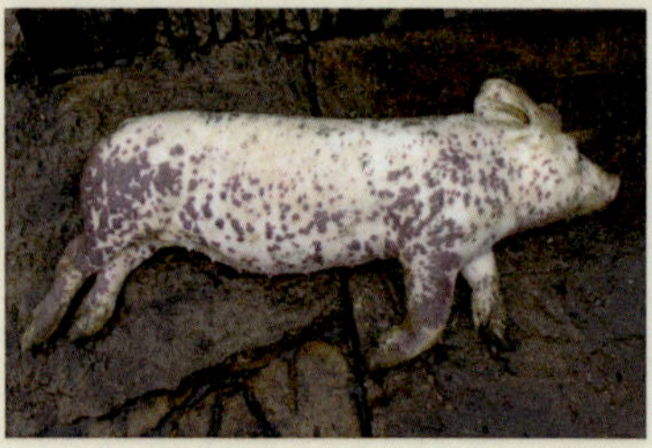

Figure 69. Porcine dermatitis and nephropathy syndrome (PDNS).

RECTAL STRICTURE

Causal agent	Stricture of the rectum leading to problems passing faeces. While the pig grows the rectal stricture does not grow, causing severe constipation.
Age group	Growing/finishing pigs.
Clinical signs	• A stricture can be felt in the rectum about 2 cm proximal to the anus. • Swollen abdomen and weight loss (Fig. 70) due to continued eating but incapacity of adequate defecation. • Eventually, the pig becomes toxic from the breakdown products being released from the stored faeces in the colon.

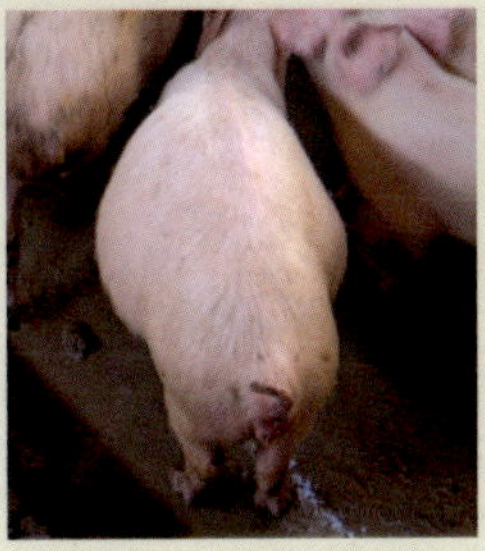

Figure 70. Appearance of a pig with rectal stricture in the grower-finisher house.

PROLAPSES

RECTAL PROLAPSE

Causal agent	Excessive abdominal straining that may be associated with a number of factors, including: • Dietary: constipation due to low fibre or water shortage). • Environmental: excessive slope to the floor, too short lying area for sows (so that their perianal region hangs over), poor condition of the floor and stocking rates leading pigs to strain when feeding or piling). • Disease-related: mycotoxins, increased abdominal pressure in case of diarrhoea, colitis or coughing. • Poor tail docking: too short docking resulting in poor anal sphincter action.
Age group	Sows (in particular around farrowing) and growing pigs.
Clinical signs	Everted mucosal tissue from the rectum protruding through the anus (Fig. 71).

VAGINAL PROLAPSE

Causal agent	Mainly management factors: • Fat sows with large litters. • Floors with excessive slope. • High feed intake and fermentable feed increasing abdominal pressure. • Stretching and relaxation of pelvic ligaments.
Age group	More common in older sows than younger, mainly over parity 5.
Clinical signs	Everted vagina protruding through the vulva.

UTERINE PROLAPSE

Age group	Sows after farrowing.
Clinical signs	• Prolapsed uterus (Fig. 72). Although it is possible to replace, the condition is generally fatal. • Most sows will die of shock (Fig. 73). Once the uterus is replaced, the high concentrations of potassium in the compromised tissues may lead to heart failure in the sow. If the sow survives replacement or amputation, she should be culled.

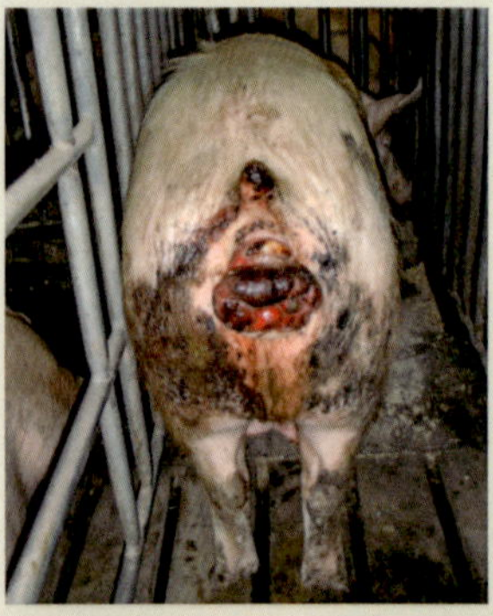

Figure 71. Prolapsed rectum in a sow.

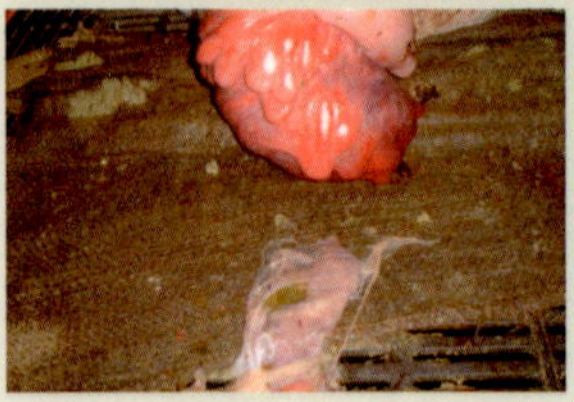

Figure 72. Prolapsed cervix.

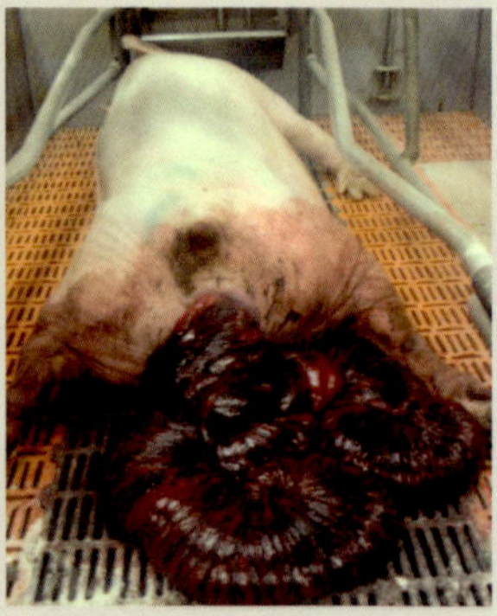

Figure 73. Postmortem view of a sow with a prolapsed uterus.

SKIN LESIONS

ERYSIPELAS

Causal agent		*Erysipelothrix rhusiopathiae*, a bacterium found on most farms. There are over 25 serotypes, however types 1 and 2 are the most common.
Age group		The disease can affect any age group. Rare in weaners below 12 weeks of age, as they are protected by maternal antibodies.
Clinical signs	Peracute	Pig found dead with no clinical signs.
	Acute	• Sudden onset. • High temperature (40–42 °C). The infected pig is often separated from the rest of the group and may appear chilled and cold (typical of a high fever). Sows may abort with the high temperature. Boars may become infertile, which may be permanent or last 6 weeks. • The pig is generally found lying down and reluctant to rise. Stiff walk, tucked up and lethargic. The pig appears to have a sore abdomen. • Off feed, sometimes constipated (young animals may have diarrhoea). • Diamond-shaped, pink to dark purple skin lesions appear 2 to 3 days later (Fig. 74). • The lesions are generally raised which may be the only way to diagnose the disease in black pigs. The skin lesions may become necrotic in the centre. The more severe the lesions, the poorer the prognosis. • Untreated pigs may die or start to recover in 4 to 7 days.
	Subacute	Diamond lesions with few other clinical signs (no loss of appetite) .
	Chronic	Two forms: • Endocarditis: The pig develops breathlessness and poor circulation especially after exertion (e.g. mating). This can result in sudden death. The pig's ears and tail may go purple with the poor circulation. • Arthritis: Three weeks after infection, the pig may present with a chronic lameness in one or two joints. It can affect the vertebrae causing the pig to have a sore back and difficulty walking.

Postmortem lesions	Peracute	Often very few lesions. Possibly an enlarged spleen.
	Acute	• Typical, often raised skin lesions. • The spleen is generally very enlarged
	Chronic-heart	Endocarditis: a "cauliflower" lesions growing on the heart valves (Fig. 75). The heart may be enlarged associated with the poor circulation.
	Chronic-arthritis	Severe arthritis in one or more joints.

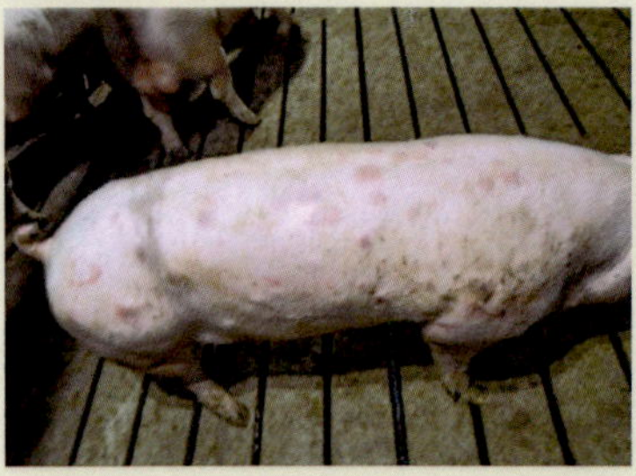

Figure 74. The classic raised diamond-shaped skin lesions of a pig with erysipelas.

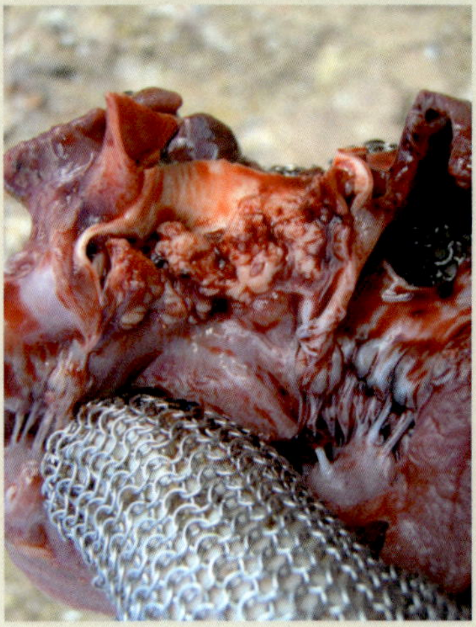

Figure 75. Postmortem lesion in a pig with endocarditis.

SKIN TRAUMA

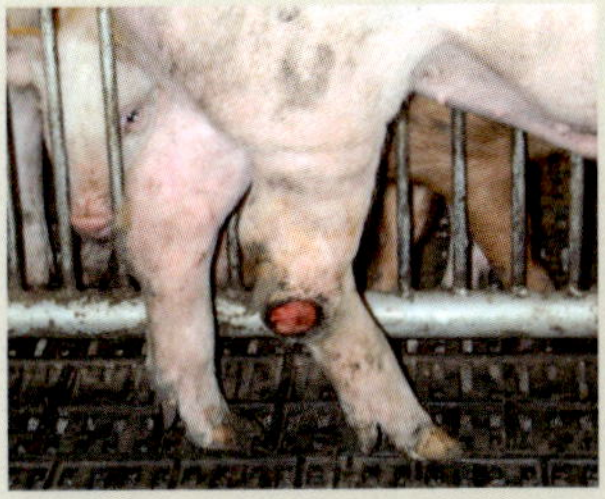

Figure 76. Tuber ulcer.

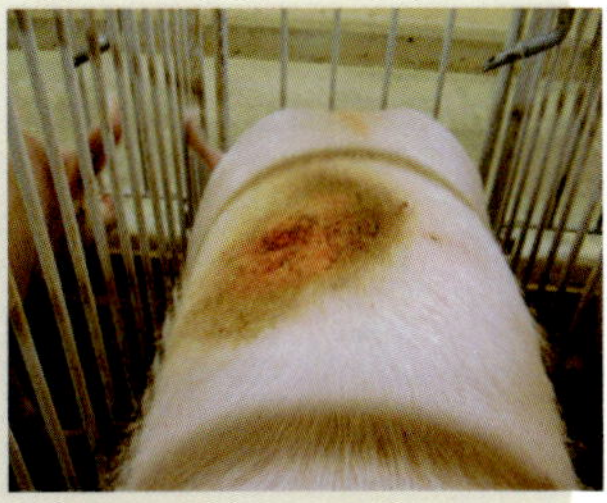

Figure 77. Housing injury.

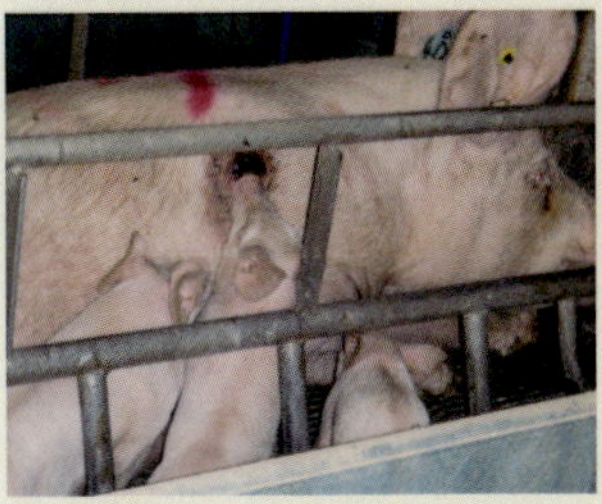

Figure 78. Shoulder sore.

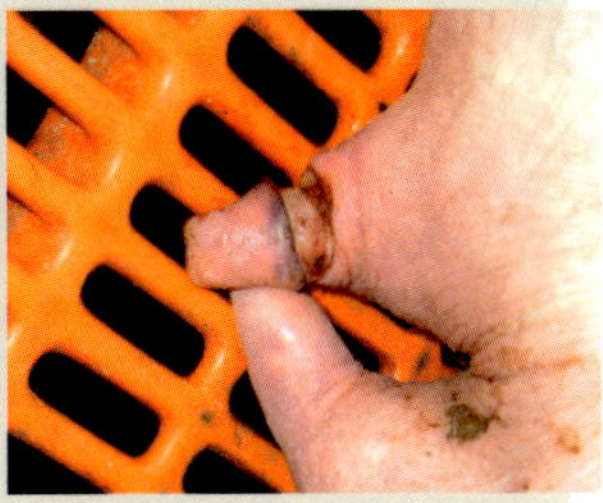

Figure 79. Teat trauma.

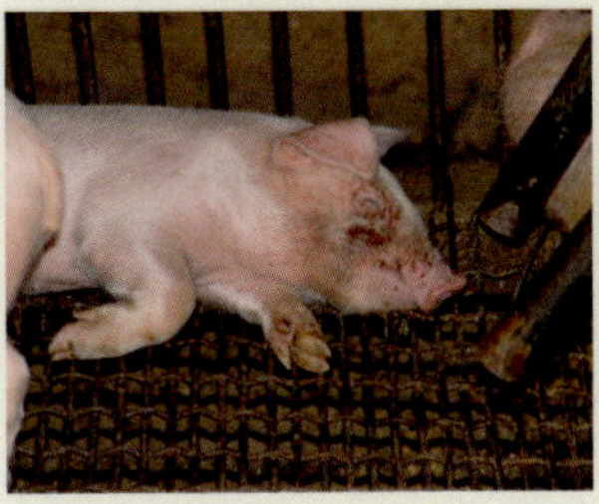

Figure 80. Facial necrosis.

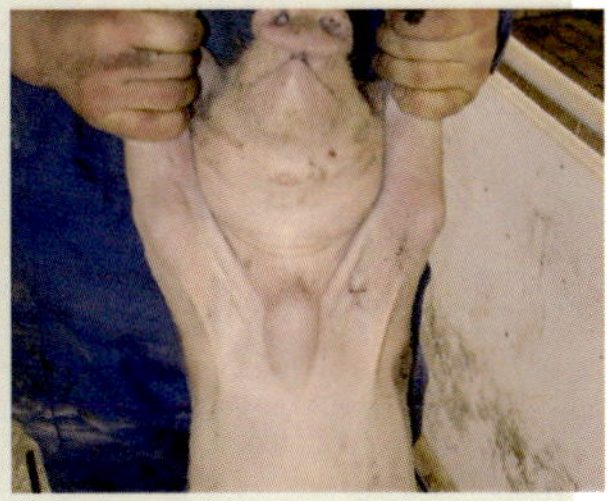

Figure 81. Bursa.

TAIL BITING AND OTHER VICES

Causal agent	Stressed and deprived pigs, often due to poor management. Check the following: • Stocking density. • Tail length, in particular variability. • Feed particle size (target> 500 μm). • Salt (NaCl) concentration in feed. Check water supplies. • For evidence of a draught at pig heights (draught air speed > 0.2 m/sec). • Air quality (target - NH_3 < 20 ppm H_2S < 10 ppm and CO_2 < 3000 ppm). • Humidity (target between 50 and 75%). • Light intensity. • Feeder space availability. • 24-hour temperature fluctuations. • Mixing pigs. Moving pigs. • In cases of facial necrosis check the milking ability of the sow.
Age group	All age groups.
Clinical signs	• Ear sucking/ear biting – in nursery pigs. • Penile sucking – newly weaned pigs (Fig. 82). • Tail biting – grow/finishing pig, rarely in adults (Fig. 83). • Flank biting – grow/finish. • Vulva biting – adult females when loosed housed (Fig. 84). • Bar biting and other stereotypies. • *Treponema pedis* may be isolated.

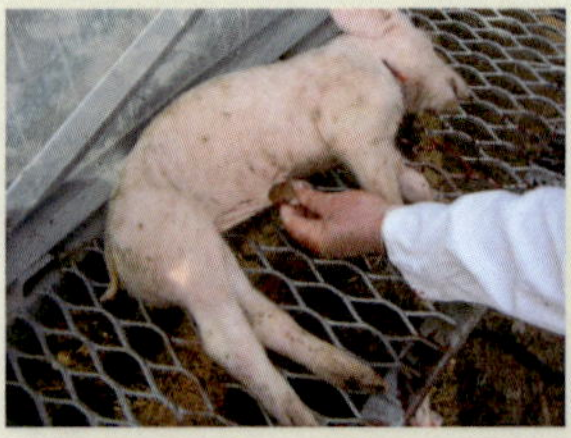

Figure 82. Penile sucking.

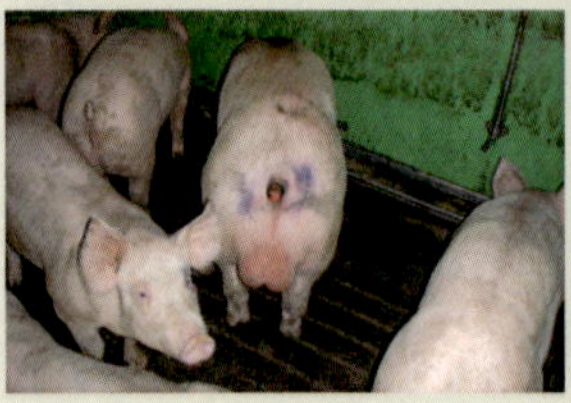

Figure 83. Tail biting.

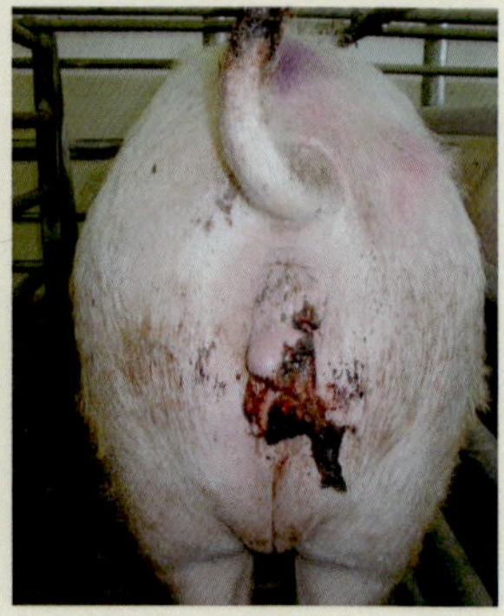

Figure 84. Vulva biting.

GREASY PIG DISEASE, EXUDATIVE EPIDERMITIS

Causal agent		*Staphylococcus hyicus*, a common bacterium colonising the skin of many pigs. Skin lesions from fighting may trigger the disease.
Age group		Young pigs (3–20 kg). A chronic form may be seen in adults. At any age, wounds that do not heal properly may have a localised region of greasy pig disease.
Clinical signs	Classic	• Newly weaned pig suddenly presents covered in patches of dirty brown greasy wet skin (Fig. 85). The hair is matted and may become a grey colour. The condition extends rapidly, covering the whole body. • The pig stops eating and drinking and becomes very dehydrated. • After a week to 10 days the pig may be found dead.
	Chronic	• Patches of 3–5 cm of "greasy pig" skin but they do not spread. • Most common/severe on the upper neck and hind legs (fight wounds).
	Piglet	Facial necrosis is a form of greasy pig disease associated with poor milk let-down resulting in excessive fighting between the piglets and damage to the face.
	Adults	A chronic black, spotty appearance on the back and neck of sows.

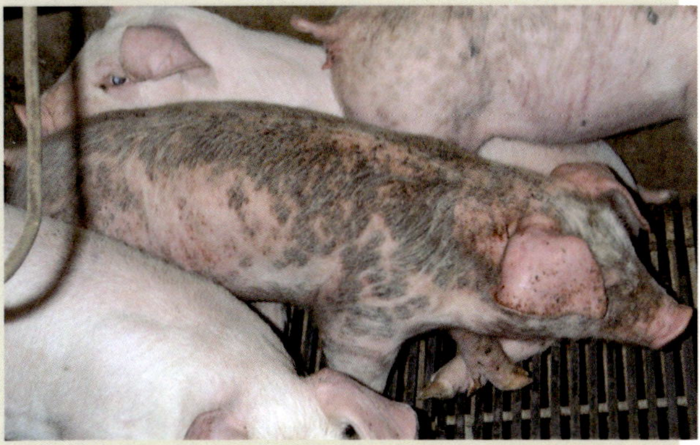

Figure 85. Patches of dirty brown greasy wet skin in a piglet with greasy skin disease.

PITYRIASIS ROSEA

Causal agent	A hereditary condition.
Age group	Young pigs (10–60 kg).
Clinical signs	• Scabby, raised, ring-shaped lesions over its body, in particular the ventral abdomen (Fig. 86). • With time the lesions may grow and coalesce. • The pig is not ill and grows normally, although looks quite alarming.
Other remarks	No treatment is necessary as the condition resolves in 6–8 weeks. The condition is rarely present by the time of slaughter. However, it is wise, not to breed from afflicted animals.

PORCINE DERMATITIS AND NEPHROPATHY SYNDROME (PDNS)

Causal agent	Unknown, suggestive of a type III hypersensitivity reaction. Porcine Circovirus 2 may play a role. Association with *Pasteurella multocida* A.
Age group	Mainly pigs from 40 to 70 kg (12 to 16 weeks of age). Occasionally in adults.
Clinical signs	Although the condition occurs sporadically on normal farms, on farms with PCV-SD it can reach a prevalence of 10 %. • Anorexia, depression, stiffened gait. Pigs lie down a lot and may have problems rising. • Irregular red to purple blotchy patches (macules and papules) on the skin, particularly around the hind legs and perineal area. The lesions tend to merge with time and if the pig survives, scarring may occur. • Pigs generally die within a few days of showing clinical signs. • Pigs affected before 10 weeks of age (30kg) will die. • In pigs older than 10 weeks, mortality may reach 25 %.
Postmortem lesions	• Both kidneys are enlarged (2–3x normal size) and pale, with cortical petechiae (Fig. 87). • Histology reveals acute glomerulonephritis and systemic necrotising vasculitis, very similar to swine fever. • Lymph nodes may be much enlarged with typical PCV-SD changes, even though the association with PCV-SD is still unclear.

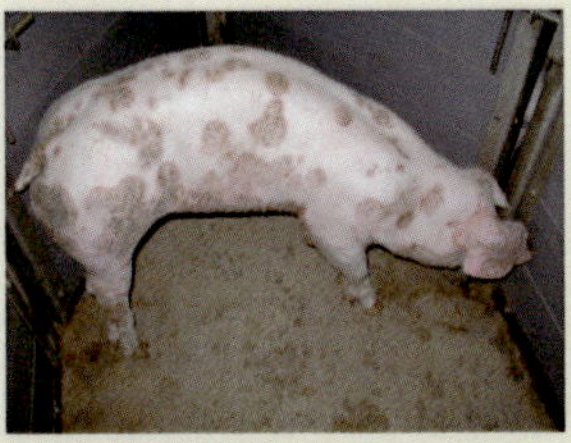

Figure 86. Scabby lesions on the ventral abdomen of a pig with pityriasis rosea.

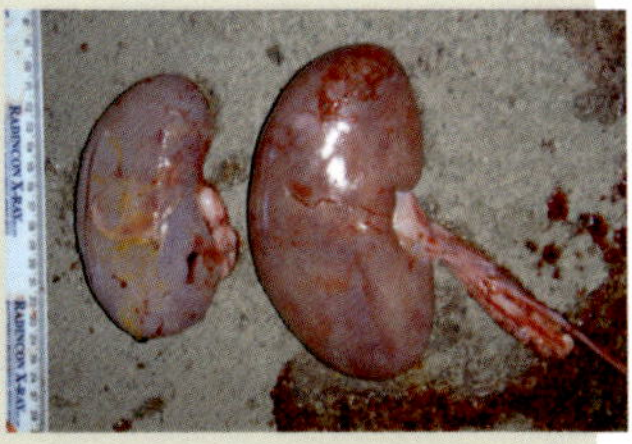

Figure 87. At left, normal kidney and at right, kidney from a pig with PDNS.

SHOULDER SORES

Causal agent	Ischaemia (lack of blood supply).
Age group	Sows in the later stages of lactation, generally in thin sows.
Clinical signs	Necrosis over the shoulder blade due to lack of blood supply.
Other remarks	• Keep the wound clean until weaning. Provide pain management as appropriate. • After weaning, place the sow in a compromised pen with straw. Feed the sow to restore body condition. • Healing is normally complete within a month. The sow should be bred as normal after weaning.

SWELLING UNDER THE SKIN

UMBILICAL HERNIA

Causal agent	A congenital defect with some genetic basis. Can occur as a major problem on pig farms.
Age group	All ages. More clearly recognised in older pigs.
Clinical signs	Large swelling under the skin in the umbilical area. In pigs over 30 kg the hernia can reach a gigantic size (Fig. 88).
Other remarks	The animal only has an economic future if the diameter stays below 30 cm and none of the skin is ulcerated. Once the hernia makes contact with the ground, euthanasia is advised. There is no economically viable treatment.

INGUINAL HERNIA

Causal agent	Very large inguinal canal (common in Vietnamese Pot-Bellied pigs).
Age group	Males.
Clinical signs	Inguinal hernias can be very large (Fig. 89). • Although rare, strangulation of a portion of the intestines can occur through the hernia. Uncastrated animals will normally grow without problems to slaughter weight. • If castration has to be performed, it should be ensured that pigs do not have a scrotal hernia. Closed castrations are advised.

ULCERATIVE GRANULOMA, ULCERATIVE SPIROCHAETOSIS

Causal agent	The spirochaete bacterium *Borrelia suis* may be a specific cause.
Age group	Sows
Clinical signs	Large granuloma on the fore or hind leg of the sow (Fig. 90). The lesion looks more severe than the behaviour of the animal would indicate.
Other remarks	There is no effective treatment. Lesion size can be controlled by housing on straw. Culling may be beneficial. The slaughterhouse veterinarian should be contacted to discuss any welfare or transportation issues before sending in the animal.

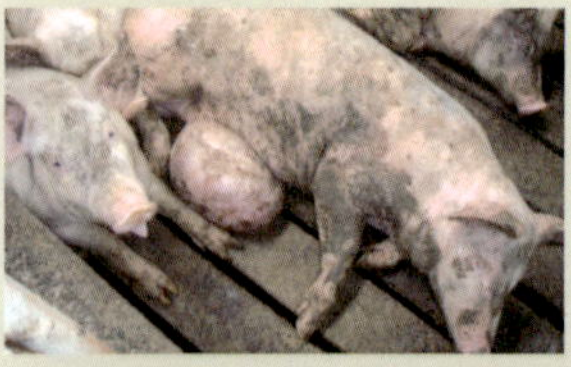

Figure 88. Gigantic size hernia.

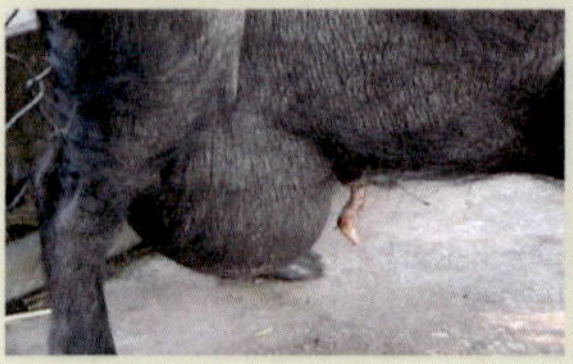

Figure 89. Inguinal hernia in a pig.

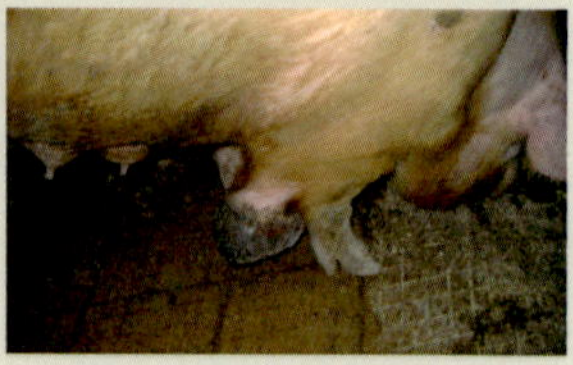

Figure 90. Ulcerated granuloma on the hind leg of a sow.

SLAUGHTERHOUSE COMPLAINTS

ASCARIS SUUM (MILK SPOT LIVER)

Causal agent	*Ascaris suum*. The adult roundworm is large (females 20–40 cm, males 15–20 cm) and may lay 2 million eggs per day. It can live 6 months.
Age group	All age groups
Clinical signs	• Clinical signs are rare, sometimes some reduction in growth rates. • Migration through the lung may result in an asthmatic cough and the pig may have problems breathing. *Ascaris* will exacerbate other lung conditions, especially swine influenza. • Young, severely infested pigs may show intestinal blockage, rupture and death.
Postmortem lesions	• White spots on the liver ("milk spot liver") develop within days of infestation (Fig. 91). However, they disappear within 25 days. • Small lesions may be seen in the lung (mainly on histology). • Adult worms may be seen in the intestine lumen (Fig. 92).

PLEURISY

Causal agent	Pathogens/foreign particles gaining access to the pleural cavity. Microorganisms end up in the pleural cavity as part of the respiratory systems defence mechanisms.
Postmortem lesions	Fibrinous adhesions between the lung lobes (visceral pleurisy) and/or the lungs and chest wall (parietal pleurisy) (Fig. 93). Lesions are healing scar tissue and are generally sterile. It is not possible to differentiate the cause of the pleurisy by the gross examination of the carcase.
Other remarks	Pleurisy seen in the slaughterhouse may have occurred at any time in the last 5 months – thus the entire life of the pig.

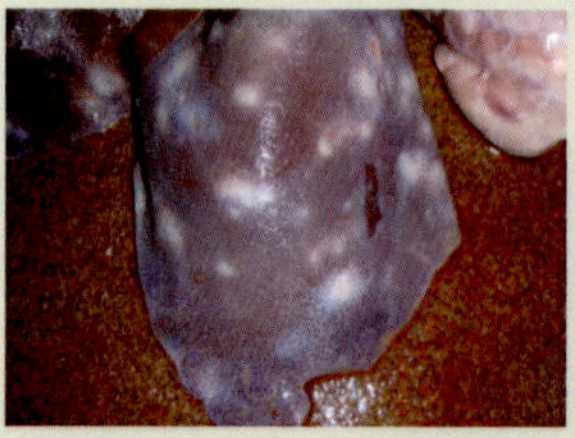

Figure 91. A severe case of white spots in the liver due to *Ascaris suum* infestation.

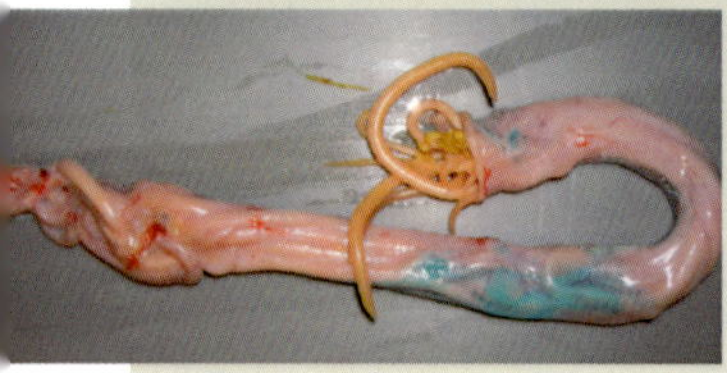

Figure 92. Heavy *A. suum* infestation in the intestine (slaughter finding).

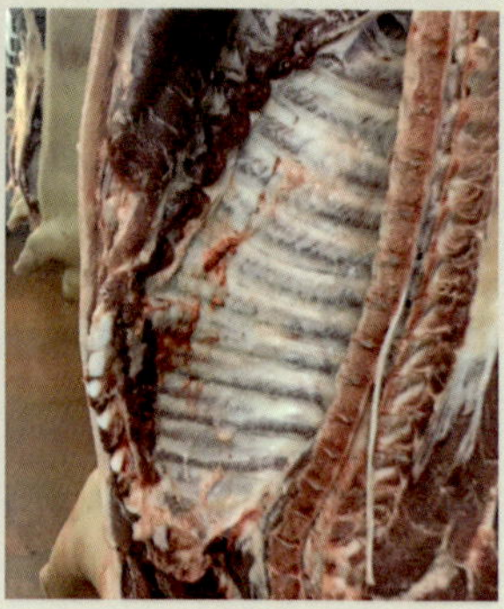

Figure 93. Parietal pleurisy seen on the surface of the lung.

SNEEZING

POSTWEANING SNEEZING

Causal agent	Multiple bacteria and viruses, including *Pasteurella multocida*, *Bordetella bronchiseptica*, *Haemophilus parasuis*, *Actinobacillus pleuropneumoniae*, *A. suis*, *Streptococcus* spp., *Pseudomonas* spp., *Proteus*, mycoplasmas, *Chlamydia*, Porcine cytomegalovirus (inclusion body rhinitis) and PRRSV.
Age group	Weaned pigs, typically 10–30 days after weaning.
Clinical signs	• Mild to severe sneezing. • The sneezing may progress to middle ear disease. • The signs progressively reduce within 2–3 weeks. • Conjunctivitis may be seen (Fig. 94) and may be severe.

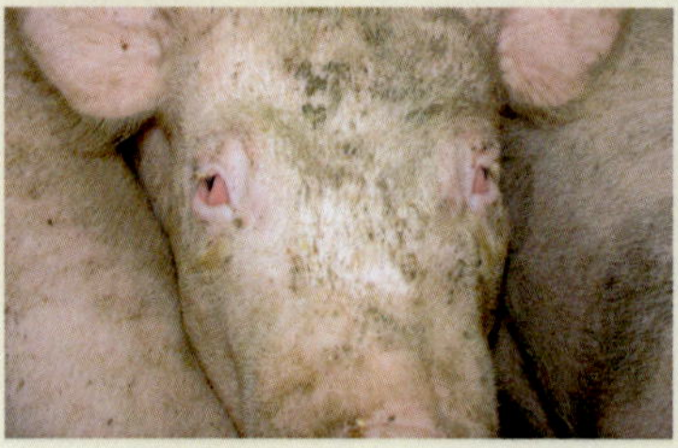

Figure 94. Conjunctivitis in a pig.

STILLBORN PIGLETS

PARVOVIRUS

Causal agent		Parvovirus, a very small DNA non-enveloped virus which makes it very resistant to disinfectants and the environment.
Age group		Only foetuses.
Clinical signs	Foetuses	The effects depend on the age of the foetus resulting in death or weakness:
Clinical signs	Foetuses	• 10–30 days of gestation: death and reabsorption – sow returns to oestrus.
Clinical signs	Foetuses	• 30–70 days of gestation: death and mummification. Bone develops after 35 days therefore reabsorption cannot occur.
Clinical signs	Foetuses	• 70–term: birth of weak piglets and mummification. After day 70, the piglet is able to mount a weak immune response to fight the disease itself but may weaken the foetus.
Clinical signs	Foetuses	The virus can move across the placenta and reach each foetus along the uterus. The foetuses die at various ages/stages of pregnancy, and therefore have a variety of crown-rump lengths (this helps to differentiate from mycotoxins).
Clinical signs	Sows	Stillbirths, mummified piglets (Fig. 95), embryonic deaths, infertility (SMEDI) and the production of a significantly reduced number of piglets born alive. Abortion is not a feature of parvovirus infections.
Other remarks		Parvovirosis is an unlikely diagnosis when there are more than 8 piglets born alive.

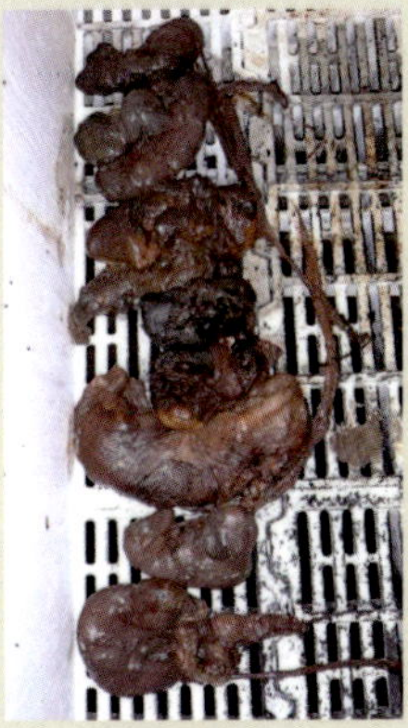

Figure 95. Mummified foetuses of variable size.

STILLBIRTHS AND MUMMIFICATIONS

70–90 % of stillborn piglets occur during farrowing. PRRSv is a major cause of prefarrowing death.

Recognising the stillborn piglet

Age at death calculated as:

$$\frac{\text{Crown-rump in mm}}{3} + 21 = \text{days of gestation}$$

In a postmortem exam the lungs will sink in water.

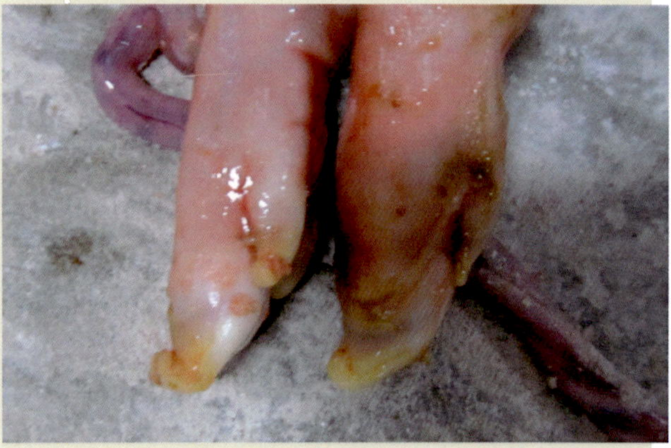

Figure 96. A stillborn piglet will still have thimbles on the toes.

REDUCING STILLBIRTHS

1	Supervision	Check the sow every 30 minutes. Use oxytocin 2.5 to 5 IU. Intravulval injection. Check the amount of prostaglandin inducement. Manual interference.
2	Age of the sow	Stillbirths increase after parity 7.
3	Increase in litter size	The number of stillbirths increases in litters of more than 12 piglets.
4	Recognise the problem sow	E.g. older sows with problems in previous litters.
5	Slow farrowings	If farrowing take longer than 8 hours, iron or calcium in the blood may be low. (Normal blood Fe > 9 µmol/l; Ca > 1.9 mmol/l).
6	Sow feeding / condition	Lack of exercise, obesity, high parasite levels or disease will increase farrowing times or result in poor uterine tone.
7	Temperature of farrowing house	Keep the environmental temperature below 22 °C. Watch placement of rear heat lamp.
8	Nutrition/water	Check the water flow rate (> 2 litres per minute) and increase dietary fibre before farrowing, as both help to reduce constipation. Do not overfeed before farrowing as this may lead to oedema.
9	Vaccination	Vaccinate gilts against parvovirus (single injection) at 6 months of age.
10	Crate design	Allow sufficient room for stockpeople to comfortably attend to the sow at farrowing time. Reduce stress and ensure sows are not cramped when lying down. No draughts. Keep lights dimmed. Playing music will help to settle sows. Intermingle sows and gilts.
11	Management of piglet tasks	Do not to clip teeth, place tattoos etc. in piglets within hearing of sows farrowing to reduce stress.
12	Feed back	Feed to gilts and sows, as this helps to stabilise the sow's immunity.